# DEMENTIA PREVENTION

A Johns Hopkins Press Health Book

# DEMENTIA PREVENTION

## Using Your Head to Save Your Brain

Emily Clionsky, MD
Mitchell Clionsky, PhD

Johns Hopkins University Press
Baltimore

**Note to the Reader:** This book is not meant to substitute for medical care, and treatment should not be based solely on its contents. Instead, treatment must be developed in a dialogue between the individual and their physician. The book has been written to help with that dialogue.

Johns Hopkins University Press
2715 North Charles Street
Baltimore, Maryland 21218
www.press.jhu.edu

Library of Congress Cataloging-in-Publication Data

Names: Clionsky, Emily, 1952– author. I Clionsky, Mitchell, 1950– author.
Title: Dementia prevention : using your head to save your brain / Emily
    Clionsky, MD, and Mitchell Clionsky, PhD.
Description: Baltimore : Johns Hopkins University Press, 2023. I Series: A
    Johns Hopkins Press health book I Includes bibliographical references
    and index.
Identifiers: LCCN 2022031479 I ISBN 9781421446240 (hardcover) I ISBN
    9781421446257 (paperback) I ISBN 9781421446264 (ebook)
Subjects: LCSH: Dementia—Prevention—Popular works. I BISAC: HEALTH &
    FITNESS / Diseases & Conditions / Alzheimer's & Dementia I MEDICAL /
    Geriatrics
Classification: LCC RC521 .C55 2023 I DDC 616.8/31—dc23/eng/20221214
LC record available at https://lccn.loc.gov/2022031479

A catalog record for this book is available from the British Library.

*Special discounts are available for bulk purchases of this book. For more
information, please contact Special Sales at specialsales@jh.edu.*

To Kathy Ross, for her patient, loving, supportive friendship over the last 50 years.

To Mitchell, the enduring and passionate love of my lifetime, who still continues to captivate, inspire, challenge, and delight me after 55 years.

And, lastly, to *Frogness*: we all still have so much left to do together!

—Emily Clionsky

To my father, a man of honesty.

To my mother, who taught me about life. And whose life taught me about dementia.

To Emily, my soulmate, who has held my heart since 1967.

—Mitchell Clionsky

# Contents

## PART III

# Where You Stand and What You Can Do about It

# DEMENTIA PREVENTION

# An Ounce of Prevention

---

*An ounce of prevention is worth a pound of cure.*

—Benjamin Franklin, 1773

Although Benjamin Franklin was writing about fire prevention in colonial Philadelphia, his wisdom endures and applies wonderfully to the field of personal health, with today's emphasis on screening and prevention highlighted by seat belt use, helmeted cycling and skiing, sunscreen, and cancer screening. What you might not know is that prevention is also the watchword for dementia, the progressive neurological decline that robs active and vibrant adults of their abilities to remember, reason, and care for themselves. Although much of the money and labor in the field of dementia research has been focused on a cure, these efforts have not resulted in any approved medications or treatments in more than 20 years. We've done the research on new drug developments, and we hate to break it to you, but there is little on the horizon in development that shows promise. Although cures for dementia appear to be unlikely at the present time, we want to let you know that dementia prevention is possible right now.

This book is about how you can reduce your risk of what we refer to as "all-cause dementia," which includes Alzheimer disease, vascular dementia, Parkinson disease, and dementias due to head trauma, alcohol abuse, and other conditions. Throughout this work, we will use the term *dementia* as a substitute for "all-cause dementia." Dementia prevention and risk reduction is not a new idea. Our research revealed a variety of research and theoretical papers extending back to the turn of the twenty-first century. But often these papers focused on only a single factor (such as exercise, weight, blood pressure, diabetes, genetics, medications, alcohol, vitamins) that were individually insufficient to make a great difference in the final outcomes assessed. Multiple-factor theories have emerged more recently, with probably the best example being from the British Lancet Commission's dementia prevention paper in 2017 (with an update and expanded content published in 2020). The 28 authors of this paper concluded that

·  dementia is *not* inevitable,

·  managing 12 medical conditions and health behaviors could reduce the cases of worldwide dementia by 40 percent(!), and

·  it is never too late and you are never too young to start this process of managing your health.

A more recent study in June 2022 analyzed the effects of these 12 medical factors in a population of close to 17,000 Americans from the Health and Retirement Study (HRS). These researchers concluded that the 12 Lancet factors "were associated with an estimated 62.4 percent of dementia cases in the US."

We agree with the Lancet Commission's finding, but we have also found several other important factors that can increase your ability to reduce your dementia risk. We will present to you a new visual model of how all of these factors fit together. Our goal is to empower you to take charge of your brain's future and reduce your chances of losing mental abilities as you age.

Wait a second, you may say. How can we be so confident in these statements? One reason is that individual areas of research have matured over the last decade and produced new evidence that points the way. But a greater reason is that we have looked more broadly at this field than most doctors have or can (and we are not boasting here!). It turns out that dementia often falls in the cracks between different medical professions. Dementia research appears in wide-ranging journals, often outside the specialty of individual health care providers. Surprisingly, there is not a distinct field of dementia and there are no "dementiologists." As we have looked at the science, we reviewed studies and opinions that span the fields of neurology, psychiatry, endocrinology, cardiology, neuropsychology, exercise physiology, internal medicine, pulmonology, sleep medicine, audiology, genomics, and translational research. We combined the findings of each of these areas into a cohesive picture that reflects the complexity of the factors that lead to dementia.

We also have the advantage of being both researchers and clinicians, being scientists and frontline practitioners. We see the effects on our patients and their families. We combine the distant view and the up-close application of the science. We understand that good health practices must be built on solid evidence, but we also appreciate that you are much more likely to apply that science to your life if it makes sense to you and you are given tools to put that knowledge into practice. A prevention plan is a start, but prevention practices must follow.

Where do we start? Many health or self-help books start with a promise to the reader. If you do these things (eat these foods, do these exercises, use these products, take these vitamins, change these habits), we *promise* that you will live longer, look better, have more success, be happier. That's the bargain. When you looked at the title of our book, *Dementia Prevention*, you probably expected the same promise from us. If you eat these foods, avoid these behaviors, do these physical or cognitive exercises, or take these supplements, you will prevent yourself from ever experiencing dementia. Unfortunately, we cannot make this promise. Dementia prevention is similar to fire prevention.

You can change the odds of having a fire, *but nobody can promise you that it will never occur*. No matter that you live in a modern steel, glass, and concrete home, with an advanced sprinkler system, rather than a 100-year-old farmhouse with wooden walls, old electrical wiring, and a faulty furnace, unforeseen forces can still burn down your house.

Take, for example, our patient Ellen. When we met her, she was 65 years old, happily married for more than 40 years to a truly wonderful man who adored her. She completed a junior college degree and had recently retired from working as a phlebotomist. Her medical history was as clean as a whistle. She had no family history of dementia, no personal history of head injury, no chronic medical problems, and no bad habits. She did everything possible to avoid dementia but still died from Alzheimer disease about 12 years later. She grew up in a warm, supportive family, with wonderful memories of family gatherings and summer vacations. She had great sisters, some close friends, and a soulmate husband who took her to every doctor's appointment, cooked their meals when she could no longer do so, insisted that they walk outside every day, and made sure that she never missed a dose of any medicine. She had tremendous energy and outlook. She recognized that she had a memory problem and hated its limitations. But she gladly undertook every test, followed every recommendation. Despite all of our interventions, consistent treatment with two dementia medicines, and living the most dementia-preventing lifestyle we could imagine, her memory and other mental abilities worsened every six months over the course of her disease. It was like watching a sharp knife drop—you could not catch it.

We will not be making you a promise, but we will commit to you the following:

1. We will give you our very best advice, the same advice that we give our patients, our friends, and our families.

2. We will base our advice on proven science or what is the most likely and scientifically sound advice. In our dementia prevention "restaurant," we will serve a sound and balanced diet of valuable medical and behavioral information rather than the flavor of the month—that titillating Internet title extolling some food, vitamin, additive, or meditation practice to make you dementia-proof.

3. We will skip discussion of the animal studies that are so many steps and years away from practice that you cannot use them and that may never prove usable. So don't look for us to discuss a dementia cure that helps genetically altered mice to better navigate a water maze after eating three times their body weight in some supplement.

4. We will explain what dementia is, dispel some myths about what it isn't, and show how it starts and progresses over time.

5. We will give you a personal Dementia Prevention Checklist that will help you take stock of your health and habits so that you can apply the contents of this book directly to your life.

6. We will discuss methods and techniques for you to use when you start to change your dementia risk.

Our book is based on a combined 70 years of professional and clinical experience in medicine and neuropsychology, on our review of thousands of studies and papers, and on our application of these principles to over 10,000 patients. We are dedicated to this field and have a passion for helping people to reduce their dementia risk and improve their lives.

Who are we? We are a husband-and-wife team consisting of a medical doctor, Emily, and a neuropsychologist, Mitchell. Emily completed residencies in internal medicine and in psychiatry. She is a diplomate of the American Board of Psychiatry and Neurology. Mitchell has been a board-certified neuropsychologist for more than 40 years. Both separately and together, we specialize in assessing individuals with cognitive decline from any cause. We run separate but overlapping practices in Springfield, Massachusetts. Together, we have evaluated and treated over 10,000 people suffering from memory and other cognitive problems.

We started working with people who already had significant memory disorders. Often, they were fairly far into their decline before they were referred, and there was little we could do except to confirm the diagnosis, offer support, and give advice to their caregivers. Gradually, over time and with the Food and Drug Administration's approval of four dementia medications, we could do more to slow the rate of decline. It also became clear that earlier diagnosis carried benefits for more ways to help our patients. We and others began to realize that many of our patients did not have typical Alzheimer disease and did not have only problems with memory.

We, and others in the field of neurology, began to look more broadly at vascular (blood vessel and circulation) and other medical problems as well as lifestyle issues. In 2007, we developed a protocol that incorporated those additional factors and created a personalized approach for each patient. This broader vision included metabolic risk factors; the status of vascular, cardiac, and renal functions; and the likelihood of disrupted breathing and oxygen availability while sleeping. We incorporated alcohol, marijuana, and tobacco use and more pointedly considered the prescription medications and over-the-counter compounds that each person took. We urged patients to increase their physical activity, cognitive stimulation, and social interaction. The combination of these factors, along with dementia medications, became what we are referring to as our Advanced Dementia Treatment protocol.

Although the cognitive levels of most of our patients were tracked by detailed neuropsychological testing, we also created a five-minute doctor's-office screening test for dementia called the Memory Orientation Screening Test, or MOST®. This brief test yielded a very reliable and valid score that we could use to follow our patients' thinking abilities in an objective and efficient way. We published four peer-reviewed studies about the MOST, and it became available widely through Quest Diagnostics under the name CogniSense™.

We compared 328 Advanced Dementia Treatment patients with 280 Standard Dementia Care patients over two years. Although both groups took the same levels of medication, the Standard group was treated by their family doctor or neurologist, whereas the Advanced group had more specific care in our practice. The Advanced group's treatment optimized their underlying medical conditions, corrected abnormal or slowed heart rates, diagnosed and treated sleep-disordered breathing and lack of oxygen, and corrected endocrine and metabolic problems. The groups were very similar in their age, education, and gender percentages.

Both groups had nearly identical average MOST scores when they were first evaluated. But, after six months, the Advanced group's average MOST score (on a 29-point scale) improved from 15 to 17.5, while the Standard group's score declined to 13.6. The group differences were statistically significant and due to chance less than 1 in 10,000 times. After one year, MOST scores for both groups remained significantly different from each other. After two years, the Advanced group remained stable and 2.5 points above their starting point, while the Standard group had declined to 3 points below their initial score, at 12, now in the moderate range of impairment. A graphic comparison of the groups is shown in figure I.1.

This was important data, suggesting that a lot more went into preserving cognition than just memory medications. We began to wonder what would happen if we started earlier, before the point of dementia. At the same time, other scientists were also looking at pre-dementia cognition, using the relatively new term *mild cognitive impairment*, or

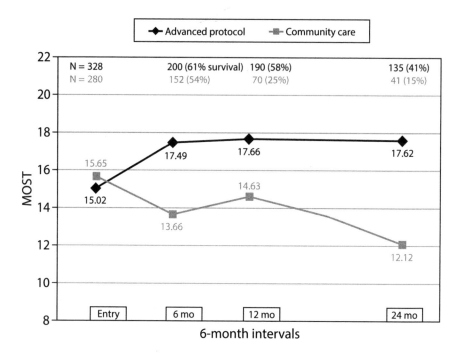

FIGURE I.1. Two-year comparison of Advanced Dementia Treatment protocol versus Standard Dementia Care

MCI. Emerging research showed that nearly everyone who experienced dementia first passed through an MCI stage, when their symptoms were mild, their everyday functioning remained intact, and they could often hide their weaknesses from others. We focused more on MCI because not everyone with MCI developed dementia. In fact, the statistics told us that only half of people with MCI declined into dementia over the next three years. We began to wonder how we could change that number, how we could keep more people from declining. We also wondered what would happen if we could start to work with them even before they had MCI.

We continued to mine the extensive database we had built on our patients. When we applied our Advanced Dementia Treatment protocol to younger people with milder levels of cognitive impairment, there were excellent outcomes.

Many individuals have remained in our practice for years (some of them now at a 15-year mark), with little change in test scores or function over this time. This is true for Allen, now 80 years old, who dutifully comes in for an annual appointment. We first met him about 13 years ago when he brought his wife in for memory evaluation. He agreed to be tested as well to make her feel comfortable but also because he forecasted that she would need to rely on him in the coming years. He was correct. And while his initial findings were fairly normal, we thought that he probably had sleep apnea and worried that his type 2 diabetes could become a problem in later years. This year, Allen remains at a level of MCI that we first saw at his third yearly evaluation. He continues to use the CPAP machine to keep his airways open that was prescribed after his positive sleep study. He has lost weight and exercises regularly, keeping his blood sugar levels in the normal range with just one oral medicine. While his wife's condition has deteriorated, he continues to provide all of her care at home, just as he had hoped.

As we saw more of the Allens of the world, we started looking even earlier at dementia prevention and discovered that dementia worry was prevalent in many people we encountered. We started to do community workshops on dementia prevention and found them to be very popular. And we learned that we could always engage the audience with the opening question, "How many of you are worried about developing dementia?" Nearly every audience member, young or old, raises a hand when we ask this question. It is not just the older people in the audience, bothered by word-finding problems and everyday forgetfulness. It is also the middle-aged and younger, often relatives of someone who has or had a dementia syndrome.

Although picking up this book would predict that you are also worried, you are not alone. Polling reveals that memory problems, including Alzheimer disease and other forms of dementia, are the biggest health concern for women over age 50. Adults of both genders over 55 report that they dread getting Alzheimer's more than any other disease, including cancer, heart disease, and all other medical conditions. A February 2022 study looking at attitudes about Aduhelm, a controversial infusion therapy for Alzheimer disease, discovered that almost 85 percent of the 1,035 people they studied were very concerned or somewhat concerned about experiencing dementia.

You are also not alone if you feel powerless to avoid dementia. Nearly half of Americans between ages 50 and 64 consider themselves at least "somewhat" likely to develop dementia. This fear permeates even the youngest of adults, at least in Great Britain, where 40 percent of 18- to 24-year-olds believe "there isn't any way to escape getting dementia as you age."

If you worry that you will get dementia and that there's nothing you can do to avoid it, we hope to change your mind. We hope to convert you from being a Dementia Worrier into becoming a Prevention Warrior.

## How to Use This Book

You will see that the book is divided into three parts. In the first part, we trace the origins of the concept of dementia and how it has been studied over the last 150 years. We also talk about normal cognitive aging and how what may be "normal" in the sense of typical may not be optimal for you.

The second part introduces a model of dementia risk, beginning with those factors that we cannot control: our genetics, our early-life experiences and traumas, our history of injury, and educational choices. Then, as the model expands, we introduce you to the factors that you can potentially control. We look at chronic medical conditions, particularly those that involve regulation of blood pressure and blood sugar. We connect this to some emerging and important areas, such as the role of oxygen levels in your brain, especially while you are asleep. We illustrate how your weight, your level of exercise, and some common habits contribute to your dementia risk and how you can modify them. We discuss some tests you should get, some prescription medicines you might not want to take, and whether drinking alcohol is good for you. We consider what happens to your brain if you are depressed, socially isolated, or unable to hear or see well.

The third part begins with asking you to complete a dementia prevention inventory, or checklist. By answering specific questions about your health and your habits, you will be able to see how you stack up against what dementia prevention research tells us is healthy or optimal. With this information, you may feel reassured or, as we suspect, you may be motivated to read the next chapters where we talk about how to improve some of your scores to change your future risk. In this section, we discuss why making change is so hard for so many of us, and we provide you with a structured method for making targeted changes. We also throw in some tricks of the trade—some methods for making difficult changes a lot easier.

We wrote this book to integrate diverse findings from highly specialized areas of research, often from fields of science where the researchers typically do not speak to one another, into one cohesive source of reliable and accurate information about conditions that affect your brain's heath. This book is based on the original scientific findings of thousands of doctors and scientists over decades. But we are not writing this book for scientists or other doctors. We are writing it for people like you. Our goal is to integrate and translate the generally obtuse, highly technical scientific literature into concepts and principles that you won't need to have a doctorate degree to decode. At the end of the book, there is a concise summary of references for each chapter, which you may find interesting. This is just to give you a starting point to access this research yourself if at some point you choose to do so. It is not intended as a comprehensive resource for what are now considered generally accepted medical facts.

We wrote this book for people like you, at all different ages and stages of life and with all risk backgrounds due to genetics, health, and lifestyle. We wrote it for people who may want to apply these ideas to their lives and perhaps make changes to improve their brain's future. As we will show you, there are a number of effective things you can do to care for your brain now and lessen your chances of losing your memory in the future.

This is not a book about dementia for those with mid-to-late-stage Alzheimer's or other significantly impairing neurodegenerative diseases. If you or your loved one has a mid-to-late-stage diagnosis, please see your doctor for the best help. Doctors can prescribe medicines that slow the course of the disease. Consult the Alzheimer's Association, which can provide caregiver support and help in planning and managing the behavior problems that often arise as the brain's functions decline. Read *The 36-Hour Day*, which has been in print for more than 40 years, is updated regularly, and still provides the most helpful how-to advice for caregivers.

As we said at the beginning of this introduction, we cannot guarantee that following our suggestions will prevent you from developing dementia. But there is a compelling case that our comprehensive and personalized approach will help stack the deck in your brain's favor. The good news is that none of these changes are too expensive, too risky, or too difficult. None are likely to cause harm. Unlike most treatments and interventions, the only side effect is better health.

This will not be a passive process. Dementia prevention requires an active approach. You may need to change your lifestyle and some of your habits. We recognize that any change is frightening as well as exciting. But, as we have said before, you are not alone. Our job is to offer an experienced helping hand and proven tools to help you take the first step and then the next steps to improve your brain's future.

So, please read on. *Stop being a Dementia Worrier. Become a Prevention Warrior.*

# PART I

## Nature and Origin of Dementia

# CHAPTER 1

# What Is Dementia?

"Is it dementia or is it Alzheimer disease?" This is the most common question asked by our patients and families. Most people are familiar with the term *Alzheimer disease*. They know Alzheimer's is something very serious and probably life-threatening, a diagnosis more dreaded than cancer for adults over 55. Although the question they are asking is specific and technical, their underlying concern is actually, "How really serious is this?" Many people don't understand the relationship between Alzheimer disease, a specific type of dementia, and dementia as an overall class of brain disease. They think that Alzheimer disease is worse than dementia. Here is a good comparison: it is like asking "is it a car or is it a Ford?" We then explain that Alzheimer disease is one of the diseases in a broader category of diseases that we call dementia. And there are actually a number of different types of dementia. Even more important, in most cases, someone has several types of dementia. We go on to explain that, no matter what type(s) of dementia someone has, the stage of their dementia is important. It generally starts with very mild disease and, unfortunately, often progresses to a more severe level over time. So, regardless of the type of dementia, one of the most important things is to discover it as early as possible.

Dementia is a progressive decline in your ability to think and act. It results in problems with your short-term memory, ability to pay attention, communication, and problem-solving. In typical cases, the most apparent loss is your ability to remember new information. While you can usually still pay attention well enough to repeat back what has just been said or to describe what has just occurred, you have much greater difficulty remembering that information after just 10 minutes or longer. It is like holding a fistful of sand in your hand—no matter how tightly you squeeze your fingers, the sand slips and slides out, leaving you nearly empty-handed. This is often frustrating and can be frightening. You try to compensate by taking notes, writing lists of things to do, and filling your wall with sticky notes. Some people keep multiple calendars or stuff their pockets and purses with reminders. Other folks seem oblivious to their memory problems, a condition called anosognosia—an inability to see that there is anything wrong with the way you are thinking or acting. Still others rationalize that they only forget things that are unimportant.

Surprisingly, while short-term memory becomes increasingly worse, long-term memory usually remains intact until much later in the disease process. As a result, many of our patients can remember who they sat next to in second grade but not what someone told them five minutes before. Those older memories were created by much younger brains that had many more connections and chemical pathways. The newer memories, by comparison, must be made by older brains with fewer cells and more limited connections.

While short-term memory loss may be the hallmark of dementia, this disease also affects a number of other mental abilities. We often see problems in someone's planning and organization skills. They can have problems staying on task or managing two or more tasks at the same time. The experienced family chef who had no problem turning out a four-course dinner for six guests now gets flummoxed trying to get all the dishes for a holiday meal on the table at the same time. A prim and proper person becomes uncharacteristically disinhibited, especially after having a glass of wine or spirits. The raconteur who always told the best stories and jokes loses track of where the story is going or forgets the punch line.

Before you hit the panic button, please understand that all of us, regardless of age or cognitive ability, sometimes forget some things. Each of us can get confused by having to do multiple jobs at the same time, especially under pressure. And even seasoned comedians can forget a punch line. Many of these occasional slips in our everyday thinking overlap with the early signs of dementia, so much so that ominous symptom checklists ("Do you have these 8 symptoms of dementia?") are poor indicators of who is really on the brink of cognitive problems.

So, back to dementia.

*Dementia* is a word much like the words *decline* or *deteriorate*. It means that the person has less mental ability than they had before. Dementia is caused by changes in brain structure, both in the outermost layer of the brain, the cortex, and in the deeper, or subcortical brain regions.

As you will read later in this book, there are many different causes for dementia. And the science is constantly evolving. Sometimes new evidence overturns the ideas that dominated the last 20 years of research. What has held firm, however, is that dementia is not a temporary condition. Dementia is also not something that a person does voluntarily. It is not for lack of trying or desire. And it is not a psychiatric disease or a type of "evil," contrary to the misspoken rhetoric of both Presidents Obama and Trump, who each publicly characterized mass murderers as "demented" individuals. Dementia is a medical disease, a neurological or neurodegenerative illness. In this book, we will most often use the general term *dementia* to highlight the fact that we are including a number of underlying medical problems and disease states.

Dementia typically begins slowly and insidiously. Evidence for Alzheimer disease biomarkers are evident years before there is any change in thinking. Changes in the end points of blood vessels are often seen on MRI (magnetic resonance imaging) scans before that person is experiencing a notable cognitive difference. Although certain events, such as a stroke, a fall, an infection, or a surgical operation, can trigger a more sudden decline in function, this rapid change typically will not occur in people whose brains are intact. The triggering event is the catalyst, the straw that breaks the camel's back, but the underlying medical process often started in early or middle adulthood. Dementia then becomes apparent when additional stress is placed on that person's cognitive reserve.

Take Helen, for example. She was a 71-year-old widow who had been living alone for the three years since her husband died. She appeared to be doing well. She continued to play mah-jongg once a week, talk with her children almost every day, pay her bills, keep up her house, and drive her car. But then she fell and broke her hip. She spent a few weeks in the hospital and a few more in a rehab facility. Then she began to show more evident confusion and forgetfulness. When it was her time to return home, her children were hesitant but hopeful that she would be more "with it" in her own environment. Unfortunately, home was now a confusing and frightening place for Helen. At her next medical appointment, her doctor administered a brief mental status examination. She did not do so well on this exam, and her subsequent MRI showed multiple areas of deterioration in underlying brain structures. This made sense, as she had been having difficulty controlling her diabetes and her blood pressure, and only recently had she been able to kick a decades-old smoking habit. Her brain scan, in this case an MRI study, also showed evidence of one or two small strokes a few years back that nobody knew about.

According to her doctor, Helen now had a mild to moderate dementia, with clear evidence of memory impairment and confusion. Her doctor said it was probably a combination of vascular dementia and Alzheimer disease. Although her hip fracture was the accelerating event, it was not the actual cause for her decline.

Just like Helen and her family, most everyone is touched by dementia. You may have seen it firsthand in your life partner, your parent, or a sibling, or maybe at a slight distance in your neighbor, friend, or an old schoolmate. Since 1 in 10 people over age 65 suffer from dementia, its effects spread outward like a ripple, touching those around them. Whatever the relationship, that person in your life who has been diagnosed with dementia has changed. That person is losing or has already lost crucial abilities to manage a job, to enjoy a hobby, and to cope with daily stresses and problems. Tragically, that person ultimately may become a confused shadow of a former competent self, unable to find the words to complete a sentence or trailing off in their thoughts. They may forget what you just told them or repeat the same stories to you. More than just misplacing their purse or keys, they may become lost while driving home from their neighborhood grocery store.

In our practice, we have heard so many of these stories. A man who went to pick up pizza at a restaurant a few blocks from home and ended up in the next state, three hours away. The mother of five who took the train to visit her adult children, changed trains along the way, and arrived without her suitcase or her purse. The frightened woman who believed that someone broke into her apartment overnight and cooked food on her stove; the crumbs and splatters she pointed to as "evidence" were the remnants of the dinner she never cleaned up the night before. We have seen formerly eloquent speakers now unable to complete a sentence, brilliant lawyers who repeat the same stock phrase three times in five minutes, and skilled physicians who can't figure out which end is up when putting on a shirt. There are truly some terrible outcomes from dementia.

It is not just memory or directional sense. People with dementia often have profound personality changes. Fastidious people become sloppy and apathetic. "Sweet little old ladies" reveal an underlying vocabulary of vulgarities that shock their children. Confident, competent elders become childlike, dependent, and afraid of someone living in their closet. In the world of dementia, we witness the profound loss of a person's defining and unique characteristics. We see the fading away of their preferences and dislikes. We observe all of the attributes that defined who they had been as a person slipping away.

Dementia is a worldwide, growing problem. Already, today, the numbers are staggering: 50 million people worldwide (diagnosed with Alzheimer's) with care costs close to 1 trillion US dollars annually. With a new case diagnosed every three seconds, dementia is projected to cost 2 trillion dollars and globally impact 82 million people by 2030 and 152 million individuals by 2050.

Why is dementia growing at this rate? The simple answer is that we are living longer. Age is the number one cause for dementia. The term *Silver Tsunami* was coined in 2005 by the Pew Research Center to describe a disproportionate increase in older people because of medical advances in longevity. By 2035, there will be more people over 65 than under 18. By 2050, approximately 20 percent of the world's population will be over 60 years old.

With longer lives come more people with dementia. In our 60s the risk of dementia is about 10 percent. This risk increases to about 25 percent in our mid-70s. And if we live into our mid-80s our risk rises to 40 percent. By 2050, when approximately 5 percent of the individuals in the world will be 85 years old or older, a tripling of elders with dementia is predicted.

While those are shocking numbers, they are only part of the story. The published data actually underestimate the true prevalence of dementia in the United States for several important reasons. First, the numbers are often based on diagnoses submitted to Medicare. But many people with dementia (in one study nearly 60%) are not diagnosed by their doctors. The same doctor who goes to great lengths to test for cholesterol, blood pressure, and blood sugar levels is likely to ignore the patient's cognition. As a result, a dementia diagnosis never enters the medical chart or the Medicare records.

Despite the existence of screening tests for cognitive problems and blood tests that can be used to make a reasonably accurate diagnosis, a December 2019 survey of American doctors in internal medicine and family practice found that 40 percent "never" or only "sometimes" felt comfortable with personally making a diagnosis of dementia.

In many cases, memory problems are overlooked until they have become severe. Our 2011 study, "Identifying Cognitive Impairment in the Annual Wellness Visit: Who Can You Trust?," published in the *Journal of Family Practice*, demonstrated that patients, family members, and even physicians have trouble detecting cognitive impairment. Although we found that a five-minute test of cognition provided a far more accurate diagnosis, health care professionals typically rely on the self-report of their patients. The problem is that the same patient who can tell you where their arm hurts or if they feel sick cannot accurately tell you if they are having a thinking or memory problem. They often minimize, deny, or are unable to recognize their decline in mental ability. The other problem is one of ageism. Still today, some doctors persist in an outdated belief that memory loss is not a disorder but just a normal part of aging, maybe what you might call "Old Timer's" disease.

The final point about the undercounting of dementia is that the published data do not include another approximately 20 percent of the elderly population with mild cognitive impairment, or MCI. MCI is a precursor or prodromal state that can precede dementia for years and typically requires standardized neuropsychological testing to diagnose correctly.

# Dementia Is Not Just Alzheimer Disease

Dementia is not a specific disease but rather a final outcome from many different diseases and medical conditions that impact the brain. And, since aging typically leads to more medical problems and chronic conditions, it makes perfect sense that older age should increase your chances of this disease.

There are many types of dementia, and Alzheimer disease is just one of them. This distinction is important not just to correct a very common misconception. The distinction allows us to look more broadly at the great number of underlying conditions that lead to dementia and which offer great opportunities for prevention. Rather than searching for an elusive and specific Alzheimer's gene or developing a medication that will eliminate a single underlying cause, we need to see a bigger picture.

The broader term *dementia* is also consistent with the most recent research findings that "pure" Alzheimer disease is found on autopsy in only about 25 percent of dementia patients, and that it coexists with other diseases in another 40 to 50 percent of cases. In fact, "mixed dementias," in which Alzheimer disease is combined with vascular dementia and, to a lesser extent, corticobasal degeneration and Lewy Body dementia, are the most common underlying pathologies that result in dementia worldwide.

# A Brief History of Alzheimer Disease

Over the past 60 years, Alzheimer disease has become as synonymous with dementia as Kleenex became with facial tissues and Xerox with photocopies. In each of these examples there is a lot more to the story than just the "brand" name.

Alzheimer disease is the neurological condition attributed to Dr. Alois Alzheimer, a German psychiatrist and neurologist, in 1910. At that time in Europe, microscopic analysis of brain tissue after autopsy was a developing and very important new area of inquiry. Scientists had created specific methods to stain these tissues so that they could see changes at the cellular level that previously were invisible.

Your healthy adult brain is made up of about 100 billion neurons, or nerve cells. If you imagine a sapling pulled from the ground in winter, you have some idea of how these neurons look. They have a cell body or stem, with an array of roots on one end and a number of tapering branches on the other. Each of these cells communicates with those around it by sending bursts of chemical messengers across a space, or synapse. These messengers leave from a branch, cross one of about 100 trillion synapses, and attach to the roots of surrounding neurons.

The classic characteristics of Alzheimer disease are the presence of amyloid plaques and neurofibrillary tangles. These plaques are composed of a waxy protein, called beta-amyloid, and the tangles are the collapsed remains and clumps of microscopically small tubules that used to be the structure supporting the inside of the neurons. These plaques and tangles destroy synaptic connections between brain cells and lead to the death of brain cells themselves. As a result, they interfere with the communication of information between the cells remaining within brain networks.

While these microscopic changes are the signature of Alzheimer disease, Dr. Alzheimer was not the first doctor to note these plaques. They were first seen on the brain autopsy of an elderly patient 14 years earlier, in 1892. In 1898, they were again described in two elderly patients who had "senile dementia." The plaques and the dementia were referred to as "senile" because the patients were elderly. Technically, this refers to anyone over age 65, just as everyone under 18 is juvenile.

During this period when doctors were beginning to use these new brain tissue handling and staining techniques, it was important for them to link their microscopic findings to clinical observations and the reports of patients and their families. In other words, they needed to connect what they saw under their microscope with how that person had functioned while alive. The neuropathology centers, where brain autopsies were conducted, became closely allied with psychiatry and neurology clinics.

In European scientific communities, this new way to investigate disease was in the spotlight and it had become fiercely competitive. The best academic appointments and financial security were the rewards for the latest discoveries. Newly created university professorships were up for grabs, and the heads of university departments were society's stars.

It was also common for doctors who identified a particular cluster of findings to have that disease or syndrome named after them. What we might today call "branding" rights was extremely common in the early 1900s, with neurological entities such as Pick disease, Binswanger syndrome, Lewy Body dementia, Creutzfeldt-Jakob disease, and, of course Alzheimer disease. Today, we rarely use this convention. It has been replaced by more descriptive medical terms, such as multiple sclerosis, or abbreviations, such as CADASIL (cerebral autosomal dominant arteriopathy with subcortical infarcts and leukoencephalopathy). But 100 years ago, your fame and fortune as a medical scientist was linked to your discovery and naming rights.

# Fischer's Disease?

Another of these early twentieth-century scientists was Dr. Oskar Fischer, a protégé of Dr. Arnold Pick, who headed the prestigious German Psychiatric Clinic in Prague. Dr. Pick is credited for identifying and describing a pathology affecting the frontal and temporal (side) areas of the brain that became known as Pick disease. In Dr. Pick's lab, Dr. Fischer performed 81 brain autopsies, 16 of which were done on individuals who died with dementia. In 12 of those, Dr. Fischer found "senile plaques," what we now know as beta-amyloid plaques. He called them "miliary foci" when he published his extensive research in 1907. He then concluded, in 1910, that these were specifically associated with senile dementia. The plaques became known as "Fischer's plaques."

Meanwhile, less than 200 miles away in Munich, at the Royal Psychiatric Hospital, the already famous Dr. Emil Kraepelin was busy at work classifying psychiatric and neurological diseases. Within his laboratory worked Dr. Franz Nissl, a neurologist and one of the greatest neuropathologists of his time.

Working in the same lab was his friend and fellow neuropathologist Dr. Alois Alzheimer. Their combined efforts allowed Dr. Alzheimer to be the first to describe neurofibrillary tangles in the brain of his female patient, Auguste Deter. Dr. Alzheimer's autopsy of her brain revealed not just the tangles but also the presence of Fischer's miliary foci, or senile plaques. However, "Auguste D" was unusual because she had begun to demonstrate moderate to severe dementia at the comparatively young age of 51. When she died at 56, she was too young to be considered senile.

So, when Dr. Kraepelin reported this case of "Alzheimer's disease" in his chapter on presenile and senile dementias in *The Handbook of Psychiatry*, he regarded it as being a "presenile dementia." He differentiated the plaques and tangles of Alzheimer disease from Fischer's "plaques" because this Alzheimer's patient began to show cognitive decline before the age of 65.

Not much was done about any of these findings for some time and, over the years, Fischer's work receded into obscurity. Until the early 1970s, the term *dementia* was used for someone who lost mental abilities after the arbitrary age of 65, while Alzheimer disease was reserved for the much less common cases of presenile dementia diagnosed in someone younger than 65. This changed in the early 1970s when there was finally enough research to demonstrate that the same disease process was occurring regardless of the patient's age. Ultimately, *Alzheimer disease* became the universal term for this type of dementia irrespective of when it began.

But regardless of whether it was called Alzheimer disease, senile dementia, or senility, little attention was paid to this disease until it impacted Evelyn Stone.

Evelyn T. and Jerome H. Stone were a financially prosperous couple, living on the Gold Coast in Chicago. Mr. Stone had a well-deserved reputation in the community as an astute businessman who pioneered the inclusion of advertising messages into packaging. He used his skills as a savvy fundraiser and board member to benefit various academic and arts-related institutions. However, none of this could help him to find answers in the medical community when his wife, Evelyn, started showing mild forgetfulness in the 1970s.

Driven by his personal experience, Mr. Stone was committed to making it better. He met with members of the National Institute of Aging (NIA) in November 1979 and began to address the overwhelming lack of knowledge, research, and caregiver support for those suffering from dementia. By March 1980, the NIA designated 13 million dollars for research targeting Alzheimer disease. Mr. Stone organized family members, researchers, physicians, and caregivers into a grass-roots volunteer group, which he incorporated as the Alzheimer's Disease and Related Disorders Association, in April 1980. The association's high visibility and superb messaging quickly heightened disease awareness. And, while the name remains as the Alzheimer's Disease and Related Disorders Association, the public knows it simply as the Alzheimer's Association. While this branding has drawn much-needed support to dementia research and care, it has fostered the mistaken notion that all dementia is Alzheimer disease.

# Everything Old Is New Again

Vascular dementia is an extremely important part of the picture. Before we thought of Alzheimer disease, most doctors and the lay public were aware of "hardening of the arteries" or arteriosclerosis. This thickening and loss of elasticity of the arteries does not only occur throughout your body, it occurs under your brain's surface in what are referred to as subcortical areas. Arteriosclerosis causes blood vessels to narrow and can decrease or completely stop the flow of blood carrying oxygen to brain tissues. Combined with atherosclerosis, the narrowing of vessels due to the buildup of plaque caused by cholesterol, these two processes are referred to as cerebrovascular disease (CVD). The reduction of blood flow due to CVD will stop brain cells from getting enough oxygen (ischemia) and result in cell injury and death. These changes cause significant earlier cognitive declines that produce mild cognitive impairment, which then often progresses to vascular dementia.

The brain-impacting effects of cerebrovascular disease were first described in 1894 by Dr. Ludwig Binswanger, a Swiss psychiatrist. He wrote of "severe atheromatosis of the arteries" appearing in the white matter of the brain. And, to make the story even juicier, it was Dr. Alzheimer who named this type of senile dementia "Binswanger's disease" in 1902. He also noted "atherosclerotic changes" on the autopsy of Auguste Deter, his famous patient. So, Dr. Alzheimer himself would hardly be surprised to find the combination of several pathologies present in the brains of those with dementia today.

The reality is that dementia is generally caused by multiple conditions and processes, with 75 to 80 percent of all autopsied cases of dementia revealing the presence of multiple primary neurodegenerative diseases. New technical developments in molecular genetics and biomarkers provide us with a greater opportunity to appreciate the overlap and similarities in their pathologic mechanisms and similarities. For your reference, an alphabetical list of the most prevalent dementias and medical conditions is included here.

| DEMENTIA TYPES | CAUSAL MEDICAL CONDITIONS |
|---|---|
| Agyrophilic grain disease (AGD) | Alcohol and polysubstance abuse |
| Alzheimer disease | Hypoxia associated with sleep apnea and COPD |
| Amyotrophic lateral sclerosis (ALS) | HIV/AIDS, tertiary syphilis |
| Cerebrovascular disease (vascular dementia) | Viral illnesses |
| Corticobasal degeneration | Metabolic derangements |
| Frontotemporal lobar degeneration (FTD) | Normal pressure hydrocephalus (NPH) |
| Huntington disease | Prion diseases: Creutzfeldt-Jakob disease |
| Lewy Body dementia (DLB) | Toxin exposures: lead, mercury, manganese |
| Parkinson disease (PD) | Traumatic brain injury, including chronic traumatic encephalopathy (CTE) |

———

Let's just recap:

- *Dementia* is a general term describing a severe enough loss of cognitive abilities to compromise someone's ability to live safely and independently.
- Dementia is not one specific disease and is not caused by one specific factor. In most cases, multiple diseases and conditions interact and contribute in different ways to the overall decline in a person's mental functioning.

· Dementia due to primary neurodegenerative diseases is not curable today. There is no "magic bullet" drug or procedure to reverse the pathological changes that have occurred.

· Earlier identification of risk factors for dementia and earlier intervention into the medical and lifestyle factors that trigger or accelerate brain decline can alter the trajectory of decline and can potentially reverse the damage before it becomes too great.

In the next chapter we will see how normal cognitive aging goes off track and starts this process.

## CHAPTER 2

# Normal Cognitive Aging

Most of us believe that cognitive decline is an inevitable outcome of aging and that a decline in mental abilities is both natural and unavoidable. Like an athlete who loses "a half step" in speed or "a few miles per hour off the fastball," both the scientific and common belief is that we become progressively less efficient in how we think and that we remember less as we grow older. We see this in the reports of brain computerized tomography (CT) or magnetic resonance imaging (MRI) scans. A neurologist will often identify brain shrinkage but then classify the findings as "normal for age." In the same way, neuropsychologists compare someone's cognitive scores with people of the same age. Although that person is thinking less well than they did 10 to 15 years before, the age comparison shows them to be at the same relative point because the average standardized mental test scores have dropped as well. Our question is whether this is healthy or just normal.

The term *normal* in science and, particularly in cognitive aging, refers to the average or typical findings. A norm is usually a statistical average of many test scores drawn from hundreds to thousands of people within the general population whose scores are believed to represent the rest of us. These people represent the full range of age, both genders, diverse races, education, occupational level, and geographical zones or countries. These people are tested during the test development stage and their scores are pooled together. With known averages and how much people vary around those averages, the "norms" are used as the yardsticks that neuropsychologists use in clinical situations. Someone coming for an evaluation takes the same tests and their scores are compared with the standards. The doctor then interprets these comparisons when deciding whether that person's cognition is impaired, and if so, to what degree and in what areas. It is this data, combined with interview information, reports from others, and review of medical records, that leads to a diagnosis, suggests treatments, and answers many other questions.

A quick look at the existing test norms will, in fact, suggest that aging makes the average person slower to process information, less attentive, more forgetful for new information, and less able to solve problems. It seems inarguable that losing cognitive ability is "normal for aging."

We decided to take a closer look to see how this phenomenon affects four major areas of brain function—attention, reasoning or "executive functions," processing speed, and memory—as we age. We relied on the published test norms for age groups from 25 to over 70, using 15 standardized neuropsychological tests that have demonstrated high reliability and accuracy as measures of thinking. This information, presented in table 2.1, is derived from the individual test manuals.

We then calculated the average of the composite "normal" test scores in each of these four areas in relation to their reference score at ages 25–29. These comparisons over the adult lifespan are shown in figure 2.1.

Notice how the curve drops as age increases. In comparison to our cognition in our late 20s, various cognitive functions decline by as little as 20 percent for attention and up to 45 percent for memory over the next 50 years. Some cognitive domains decline more gradually and others more sharply, but the average score from every test we examined was higher at age 25 than at 75.

**TABLE 2.1.  Standardized Tests of Cognition**

| ATTENTION | PROCESSING SPEED |
|---|---|
| Wechsler Adult Intelligence Scale (WAIS-IV) Digit Span | Wechsler Adult Intelligence Scale (WAIS-IV) Coding |
| Trailmaking A | Symbol Digit Modalities Test |
| Stroop Word Reading | |
| Stroop Color Naming | |
| **REASONING / EXECUTIVE FUNCTION** | **MEMORY** |
| Trailmaking B | Rey Auditory Verbal Learning Test |
| Wechsler Adult Intelligence Scale (WAIS-IV) Matrix Reasoning | Trial 1 |
| | Trial 5 |
| Category Test | Recall |
| Stroop Color-Word Interference | Wechsler Memory Scale (WMS-IV) |
| | Logical Memory–delayed |
| | Visual Reproduction–recall |

To get a more general appreciation of this effect, we combined all four areas into a global measure of cognition and examined the scores over each epoch of adult life. As you see in figure 2.2, the conclusion seems the same: "Normal" performance declines as age increases. Everyone loses out over time.

This brings us to the question of what we consider to be abnormal. Abnormal is defined as test scores representing underlying mental functions in which the decline is greater than the expected rate, accounting for errors in measurement. In most cases of eventual dementia, the affected person begins to have greater than normal declines starting as early as midlife. Often, the changes are subjectively

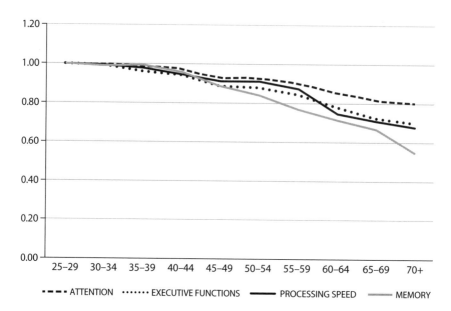

FIGURE 2.1. "Normal" test scores in attention, executive functions, processing speed, and memory decline as we age

felt by the person in their 40s and more objectively seen when they are in their 50s. Using the previous graph as the comparison point, we can show this deviation from normal in figure 2.3.

When this departure from normal first occurs, a person experiences what we call mild cognitive impairment (MCI). The thinking problems in this period are fairly mild and often not noticeable to most others.

Such was the situation with Lavinia. At age 55 she was working as a claim supervisor for an insurance company. She had been with the same employer for 25 years and had worked her way up through jobs as a clerk, adjuster, and senior adjuster. Now she supervised others and was responsible for making critical claims payment or denial decisions. While those decisions had been easy at first, she now noticed that she was less decisive and more easily drawn off task. She asked her subor-

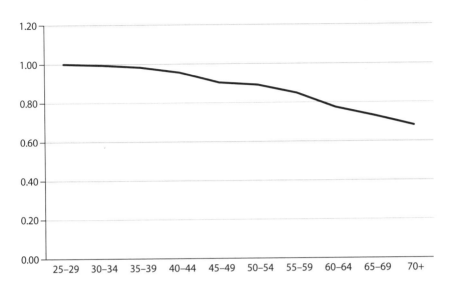

FIGURE 2.2. Global decline in brain function from 25 to 70+ years old

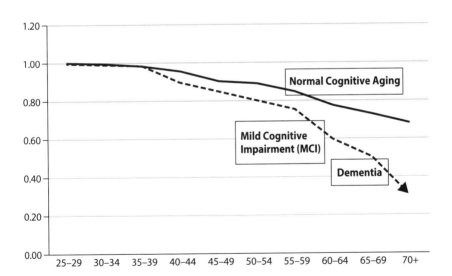

FIGURE 2.3. Decreased brain function seen in mild cognitive impairment (MCI) and dementia compared with normal cognitive aging

dinates to send her emails rather than call her on the phone because she often forgot the telephone discussion and wanted time to review each decision. She was making reminder lists, even for tasks that she had done for years. Any change to the computer system now filled her with fear. As testing in our office demonstrated, she was processing more slowly than expected, had a "flatter" learning curve, and experienced greater problems remembering new information. But, like other people with MCI, she could still do all of her everyday tasks. She had no problems driving, using an ATM, shopping online, and cooking. She did have some of the anxiety common to people with MCI who perceive that they are slipping and don't know what to do.

At the point of MCI, others may also start to see some problems. We view MCI as a wake-up call. We are always happy to see people who come in at this time because many have not yet lost abilities that cannot be recovered. But it is an alarm clock for becoming more active. Research tells us that MCI triples the risk of dementia and that 50 percent of people with MCI will decline into dementia over the next three years if nothing is done. Our goal is to stabilize the decline and look for ways to keep that person in the 50 percent who remain stable or actually improve.

The first step in this process often involves additional testing.

## Physical and Biological Markers of Cognitive Aging

Biomarkers and modern imaging techniques allow us to visualize some of the early changes in brain structure that cause dementia in the future. We no longer have to wait until death to look at the very small cell and network changes on autopsy. We can measure the activity of neural networks through functional magnetic resonance imaging (fMRI), and we can estimate the level of beta-amyloid plaque buildup through specific positron emission tomography (PET) markers. Most recently, we are seeing blood tests that measure amyloid and tau proteins in blood samples, well before a person is symptomatic. These various techniques tell us that the cognitive declines thought to be due to "normal aging" are actually directly due to pathology. However, while these reflect some of the brain changes pertinent to Alzheimer disease, they do not correlate with actual risk of eventual dementia and they overlook the greater majority of cases that involve vascular and other pathologies. To look at the vascular problems, we currently turn to MRI scans, which can identify and locate areas of damage within the "white matter" or subcortical areas of the brain.

You may have heard about white matter changes if you have had an MRI scan of your brain. The term *white matter* refers to the visual appearance of the cells in the subcortical (below the cortex or outer brain surface) areas. These cells have very long branches or projections called axons that are covered by a light-colored sheath composed of myelin. Comprised of proteins and phospholipids, this myelin coating acts sort of like the insulation on an electric cord. Myelin allows axons to transmit impulses extremely quickly, as much as 60 times as fast as those on the surface of the brain where cells have much shorter axons and are not myelinated. Those cortical axons appear gray in color (we refer to this as the "gray matter"). Using magnetic resonance imaging (MRI) scans, the subcortical white matter becomes intense or "lights up." This brightness is the result of damage or death to brain cells, largely caused by vascular diseases. When blood cannot get to the narrowest ends of blood vessels, called capillaries, white matter brain cells are starved for the oxygen that is carried by the blood and are damaged.

By the time we can detect these white matter hyperintensities on MRI, many years of injury to many different brain cells and blood vessels have occurred. It typically begins fairly early in life, before any obvious problems are noticed, and is evident on brain MRIs in as many as half of people still in their 40s. In the case of familial Alzheimer disease, the white matter changes actually start earlier, by about six years on average, and are present before memory changes and other symptoms begin to surface.

## Reexamining Normal Cognitive Aging

It seems pretty depressing, doesn't it? Cognitive test scores decline as we get older, brain volumes shrink, white matter deteriorates, and amyloid and tau proteins accumulate. From our 20s on, accelerating during our 50s and progressing thereafter, a normal person experiences physical changes in the brain and gets progressively less able to think.

But, suppose normal cognitive aging isn't so normal. Or at least not so healthy. Consider that, when each of the standard cognitive tests were "normed," the scores were derived from people in the general population. Many different kinds of people. People with underlying medical problems, people with several undiagnosed concussions from soccer or football during high school, people with diverse genetic risks and possibly poor early-life experiences, people whose mothers smoked during pregnancy or skipped prenatal vitamins. Some of these people were probably in good shape but others were not. We know that some test developers will separate out or avoid including people who have major neurological conditions, such as stroke, brain tumors, or diagnosed dementia. They will exclude people with intellectual disabilities and possibly major psychiatric conditions. However, the standard test norms in current use do not consider factors such as cigarette smoking, obesity, alcohol use levels, or reliance on benzodiazepines. These norms do not ask about or group people according to medical conditions such as hypertension, diabetes, high cholesterol, or sleep apnea. None of these norms look at subtle hearing or visual impairment, use of anticholinergic medications, current level of cognitive activity, or emotional factors of depression and anxiety.

And yet, as you will see in the coming chapters, each of these medical and lifestyle factors plays a role in how our brains work and how we think. These factors, individually and in combination, impact our risk of later dementia. As a result, our current test "norms" reflect the abilities of typical or "normal" but not optimally healthy individuals. And, since the number of medical problems increases as we get older and cumulative effects of lifestyle become more evident on our health over the long term, is it any wonder that cognitive functions decline as we age?

## The Future of Normal Cognitive Aging

So, what do we do with this information? We could throw out current cognitive testing and just rely on physical biomarkers. But neither overall brain volume changes nor shrinkage of more specific areas of the brain accurately predicts dementia. Conversely, many people die with autopsy evidence of beta-amyloid plaques, Lewy bodies, neurofibrillary tangles, and white matter changes, even while they are fully functional in their thinking right up to the end. Studies using newer biomarkers are being done in various research settings by members of the Alzheimer's Disease Neuroimaging Initiative (ADNI). However, the ADNI focus is primarily on neuroimaging markers rather than medical conditions and lifestyle factors, which are very important.

A second approach would be to conduct a super-normative study of cognition in which thousands of adults would be tested and very precise measurements of their health and lifestyle recorded. A very expensive and time-intensive approach, this would essentially expand on the model used by the Framingham Heart Study, where many cohorts of people living in eastern Massachusetts have been followed for years and their cardiac and health conditions are associated with their cognitive function. Such research data are very valuable but do not change the test scores we use.

A third approach might be to identify super healthy individuals. We could norm tests on people selected for their clean genetic profiles, excellent health, strong educational background, cognitively challenging pursuits, and healthy lifestyle habits. Then we could truly answer the question of what happens to our brains and our thinking abilities as we age. But, in doing so, we would clinically diagnose very high percentages of people with some form of cognitive impairment, even though they were living fully functional lives. Putting aside the problem of how to find a lot of these super healthy people, we do not get much closer to the question of how to help all of the rest of us, we less perfect individuals.

We conclude that we should continue to use our standard cognitive tests in clinical situations but recognize that comparing people to established norms may not do justice to some people with early cognitive concerns. Furthermore, some of the people who we think are intact may actually have mild cognitive impairment. We can reassure them that their test scores are in line with others of their age and background but may not be as good as they could be.

We believe that we should not accept a loss of mental functioning as inevitable as we age. Instead, we should do whatever we can to control our personal factors that lead to mental decline. This is certainly achievable. As of today, 40 percent of people over age 95 and 25 percent of those over 100 appear to have intact cognitive ability. We do not believe that this is just luck. While we can all hope to end up alive at those ages and to be in the group with preserved cognition, we advocate a more active approach in which we identify and control medical problems and lifestyle choices to tilt the odds in our favor. We believe that this approach is our best chance of continuing to think and remember as well in old age as we did when we were young.

Is this naïve optimism? You can be the judge as you read on. But remember the Greek fable. When Pandora opened a jar left in her care, there emerged many evils, including sickness and death. And as she tried to close the jar, there was only one thing that remained. And that was hope.

———

In the next part, you will see the progressive construction of our model for dementia risk and the factors directly and indirectly affecting a person's risk and what they can do to prevent it. This is not the only model that has been proposed, but we believe that it will give you a framework to best understand the current knowledge. This model will not include every idea that has been proposed, but rather those that we believe make sense and are backed by science.

# PART II

---

# Dementia Risk Model

---

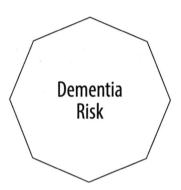

Dementia
Risk

## CHAPTER 3

# Genetics and Early-Life Factors

In the beginning, when your father's sperm encountered your mother's ovum, the point of your conception, you became a genetically unique individual. While entirely out of your control (after all, you can't choose your parents), this moment of conception determined much of who you would become. This moment determined your birth sex; your blood type; the color of your skin, eyes, and hair; and your facial features. It also laid down genetic starting points or predispositions for particular illnesses and even some of your behavioral tendencies that would later impact your dementia risk.

Understanding genetic factors begins by appreciating that every one of your 30 trillion cells contains chromosomes, which are thread-like proteins that contain the genetic code that makes you unique. These chromosomes are made up of DNA, or deoxyribonucleic acid. DNA is often called the "building block of life." It uses sequences of just four chemical codes to produce all the proteins that make up everything in your body. Amazingly, genetics tells us that as much as each of us is unique, we actually share about 99.9 percent of our genetic information with each other. Genetic variations we inherit from our parents are responsible for the remaining 0.1 percent that makes us unique. But even so, that one-tenth of a percent is very powerful.

We are now aware that even a single change in one gene can cause disease. This relatively recent finding has opened the door to a host of possible treatments or even cures. However, it is not so simple. We also know that your genes interact with each other and that your DNA and chromosomes are modified and change over your lifetime in response to your environment, socioeconomic factors, nutrition, level of stress, physical and emotional trauma, and education. These effects begin prenatally and continue throughout your life. The exact mechanism of these complex interactions and permutations is not yet completely understood, but genomics—the more formal name for this area of inquiry—is a rapidly expanding area of science. This knowledge is critical to "precision medicine," the ability to provide personalized or tailored medical care based on an individual's genetic makeup.

Although precision medicine is increasingly being used to treat many types of cancers, our knowledge is not sufficiently mature to apply this kind of precision to any specific form of dementia.

To appreciate how these genetic variations occur, let's remember that each of us has two alleles or copies of each gene, one coming from each parent. And each of these contains 23 chromosomes, labeled 1 through 22 with the last pair, $X$ and $Y$, referred to as the sex chromosomes. If you are female, you have two $X$s. If you are male, you have one $X$ and one $Y$. As a substantial number of studies have confirmed, sex matters, especially in determining our risk for dementia, with the two greatest risk factors being advanced age and being female.

Women make up two-thirds of diagnosed cases of all-cause dementia in the United States and Europe. Previously attributed only to their having a longer life span, we now know that it is a woman's hormonal status, specifically estrogen-deficient states, that results in measurable brain changes that increase her dementia risk. Estrogen deficiency reduces her ability to metabolize glucose, increases the deposition of beta-amyloid protein, and causes greater loss of brain cells in parts of her brain that have high concentrations of estrogen receptors. These overlap with regions involved in dementia, such as the hippocampus and frontal cortex. Research also indicates that cardiovascular risk factors are highly correlated with increased dementia risk and that estrogen influences blood pressure. Premenopausal females with high estrogen levels have lower blood pressures than similarly aged males due to greater expansion of blood vessels that reduces the pressure within them. Women most often have lower blood pressures (and reduced cardiovascular risk) throughout middle-age, regardless of ethnicity. But after menopause, now at an average age of 51.4 in the United States, women's blood pressures rise to levels higher than those of men, placing them at greater risk.

Women also have double the rate of depression than men, creating a second independent risk factor for developing coronary artery disease. Both depression and cardiovascular disease are closely correlated with increased rates of all-cause dementia, and this risk is independent of ethnicity and other medical conditions. These are just a few examples of how one genetic determinant, set down at conception and outside of our control, can have far-reaching effects on our brain, either directly through changes in hormone availability in the brain or by increasing our susceptibility to other medical conditions that cause eventual damage to our brain.

We also know that some specific genetic variants increase the risk of Alzheimer disease specifically. The most well-studied has been Apolipoprotein E (*APOE*), a gene on chromosome 19 that is involved in the metabolism of fats in the body and is implicated in heart and cardiovascular disease. It has several variants, $\epsilon$ or Epsilon 2, 3, and 4. From a dementia perspective, *APOE* $\epsilon$4 confers an increased risk (91%) for the development of Alzheimer disease. If you have inherited two *APOE* $\epsilon$4 alleles, one from each biological parent, not only is your risk higher but the average age of onset drops from 84 to 68. Fortunately, this double whammy occurs only in about 2 to 3 percent of the population and is somewhat offset by the rare although fortunate people who have an *APOE* ε2 allele that can reduce the typical risk by 20 percent. Most often you will have one or two copies of *APOE* ε3, which does not change risk.

The *APOE* ε4 allele also increases our dementia susceptibility in less direct but understandable ways. This allele doubles the risk of sleep-disordered breathing, particularly sleep apnea, which is known to cause cognitive impairments as well as mood disorders. Incidentally, postmenopausal women who carried this allele had a five times greater risk of cognitive impairment in the setting of obstructive sleep apnea (OSA).

Dementia genetics is not just about *APOE*. The *MTHFR* gene creates the genetic program for a critical enzyme that metabolizes and uses folic acid (vitamin B9) and cobalamin (vitamin B12). These B vitamins are essential in producing ATP, the energy molecule all of our cells need to remain alive and function properly. One single exchange of an element on the *MTHFR* gene prevents your body from using folic acid and B12, no matter how many beans, peas, and leafy vegetables you eat. And, without sufficient B vitamin levels, your brain will not work properly.

Other mutations, such as those in the amyloid precursor protein (*APP*), presenilin 1 (*PSEN1*), and presenilin 2 (*PSEN2*) genes, which influence the production of beta-amyloid, are associated with dominantly inherited forms of early-onset Alzheimer disease. In these early-onset varieties, someone can begin to experience dementia symptoms as young as in their 30s and 40s. Even so, over 90 percent of Alzheimer disease and most other types of dementia are what we call "sporadic," which means that a combination of genetic and environmental risk factors that are not yet fully understood caused the disease.

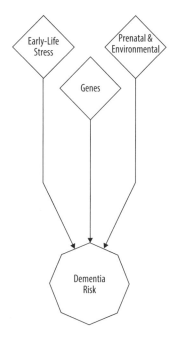

## Moving Beyond Genetics

Combined with the genetic code laid down at conception, there are events and conditions that may have occurred prenatally and in your early childhood that can also impact your cognition in later life.

What your mother ate, drank, smoked, ingested for pleasure, or took by prescription while you were in the womb can play an important part in your dementia risk. For instance, maternal obesity, at the time of conception, may start you off on the wrong foot. Research has found that greater body mass index in a mother prior to conception correlates with her child's decreased cognitive scores in primary school, independent of other intrauterine and social factors. When you consider that lower cognitive test scores in early life increase your risk of mortality up to age 76, the implications of maternal obesity become clear to anyone planning to have children. Maternal smoking, alcohol consumption, recreational drug use, and some prescription drugs also impair achievement levels in their children and create increased risk for dementia in later life.

Early-life experiences also interact with our genes to influence our children's levels of cognition and their later-life abilities. Remember those DNA strands? At the ends of our DNA strands are structures called telomeres. Like those little plastic aglets at the end of our shoelaces, telomeres protect our chromosomes from unraveling and losing genetic material whenever cells replicate or make copies of themselves throughout our lifetime. Depending on the type of cell in the human body, a telomere will last through 50 to 100 DNA replications. Once it is gone, the integrity of the DNA duplication process is compromised. We now know that children who have been subjected to early-life adversity—physical, emotional, or sexual abuse or assault; neglect; and chronic poverty—have shorter telomeres and lower cognitive scores in childhood. Shorter telomere length has been associated with earlier onset of cognitive impairment, as well as increased rates of immunological disorders, cancer, and early death.

The good news is that early-life cognitive enrichment demonstrates the opposite outcome, namely higher cognitive scores, slower onset of age-related cognitive decline, and fewer neuropathological lesions in the brain on autopsy. As you read this, you may be reflecting on your own childhood, either impoverished or enriched, and wish that you could get a do-over. Take heart that some of these factors may still be modifiable but also pay attention if you are still within childbearing or child raising age, as all of this information may help you create a better future for your child.

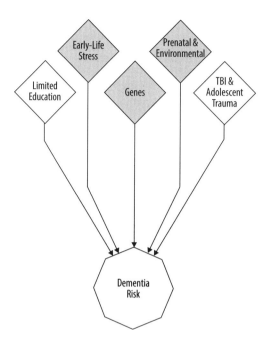

## Childhood and Adolescent Factors

To say that the relationship between our genes and all the events that transpire in our lives is complicated is obviously an understatement. Let's take a look at what happens up through our 20s.

Traumatic brain injury (TBI) has its highest peaks in early childhood and old age. It often occurs accidentally, although the greatest early childhood risk is due to child abuse. As we move into adolescence, brain injury from reckless behavior, sports exposure, and simple accidental injury becomes much more prominent. Head injuries also interact with genetic risk. Research has demonstrated that children with an *APOE* ε4 allele who also experience a mild or more serious TBI have a significantly elevated risk of poor outcomes than either those who just have the allele or who have had a head injury without that allele. The mechanisms are complicated and have to do with increased oxidative stress, a cascade of cell messengers that induce cell death, and impaired cellular repair mechanisms, all implicating the €4 allele. Thirty years of scientific study reveals that even one TBI significantly increases the risk of dementia later in life, with an escalation in probability directly linked to the severity of the injury.

More recent questions have arisen concerning the role of repeated but less severe traumas to the brain, as are found in many contact sports. When spread across a lifetime of repeated exposure, these injuries may trigger the excessive release of tau proteins to create a dementia variant known as chronic traumatic encephalopathy (CTE). This research is also complex and still a work in progress. Whether we believe that such repeated sports or other concussions are minor, tran- sitory, and ultimately resolving or whether we believe that up to 20 percent of people with concussions are never the same, we can all agree that prevention or minimization of concussions is an important goal.

Genetics also changes our risk for dementia by increasing the like- lihood of related chronic medical conditions, such as type 2 diabetes and cardiovascular disease (CVD). Most diabetes, and the early stage of insulin resistance that precedes it, has a genetic element that inter- acts with family and lifestyle factors, such as diet and exercise. Type 2 diabetes is associated with two to four times an increased risk of CVD. Either condition, diabetes or cardiovascular disease alone, is known to significantly increase our risk of developing all-cause dementia. We will be going into those factors in detail in upcoming chapters.

While genes, prenatal factors, and early-life experience are not our destiny, they are our baseline, our starting point. A recent large-scale study determined that a "favorable" lifestyle was associated with lower dementia risk for those with a high genetic propensity. Knowing your genetic baseline and the prevalence of chronic illness in your blood rel- atives (especially your parents and members of their generation and those before them) may help you to appreciate where some of your strengths and weaknesses lie. But, in doing so, and especially when considering dementia risk, recognize the probabilities. If you have one parent with dementia that began in their late 70s and they have four siblings in good cognitive health, your risk is probably no greater than anyone else's. At this time, there is no benefit to getting tested for genes associated with family-inherited forms of dementia. Without our having a disease-modifying treatment for genetically transmitted neurodegenerative dementias, your dementia prevention plan will remain the same. You will do all that you can to improve your chances going forward. You may also want to pass on genetic testing at the present time because of uncertainty about how the results of these genetic tests might be used by insurance companies in assigning risk or offering coverage. On the other hand, if you have a strong family history of early-onset cognitive loss, consider enrolling in a randomized controlled trial for an experimental treatment (see www.clinicaltrials.gov, and enter "dementia").

Our genes are our starting point. For the most part, they do not necessarily represent fatal inevitabilities. By understanding our familial inheritance and considering the pluses and minuses of our early childhood experiences, we can better plan the steps we need to take now to optimize our chances of improved brain health in our future.

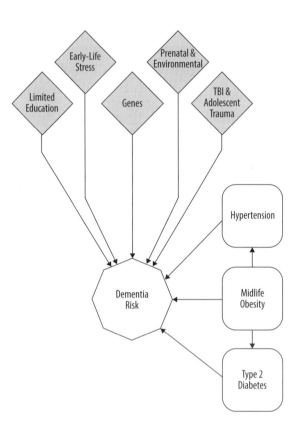

CHAPTER 4

# Midlife Medical Conditions That Affect Dementia Risk

---

By the time we reach our 30s and 40s, the initial negative effects of our genes, prenatal and early-life exposures, educational limitations, and risk-taking behaviors are often compounded by vascular and metabolic medical conditions. Based on large observational studies, the 2020 Lancet International Commission on Dementia Prevention, Intervention and Care attributed 40 percent of all dementia cases to 12 preventable risk factors. Of these, three—hypertension, diabetes, and obesity—are strongly related to each other and each, individually and in combination, impacts your cardiovascular system directly. In fact, each factor triggers a cascade of cellular injury that, over time, results in eventual damage to your brain in later life. One such type of injury involves decreased blood supply to and throughout the brain's blood vessels.

## Cerebrovascular Diseases

The blood supply to the brain is like a tree, with big arteries at the base of the brain, which branch out and become progressively smaller and narrower as they penetrate into deeper brain tissues. Eventually, this 400-mile network of microscopically small capillaries becomes so narrow that only a single red blood cell can reach a brain cell at one time. Each of these single red blood cells carries oxygen and nutrients essential for brain cells to work.

Multiple studies have found that decreased cerebral blood flow occurs early in dementia, well before someone demonstrates problems in solving test problems or a doctor can recognize tissue loss or brain atrophy on an MRI. And, when the blood flow diminishes substantially to a part of the brain, you are likely to experience a cerebrovascular accident (CVA), commonly called a stroke. Even when such an event lasts less than 24 hours and is termed a transient ischemic attack (TIA), the consequences are serious. Strokes require immediate medical care and often result in death or disability. But even for those who survive, about one-third develop dementia within three months. Overall, studies have found dementia occurs eight to nine times more often in someone who has had a stroke when compared to people who have not. High blood pressure, elevated cholesterol levels, obesity, and diabetes are just a few of the medical conditions that contribute to stroke risk, and all are modifiable.

Other cardiac events can also impact blood flow and impair nutrient and oxygen availability in the brain. When your heart loses its contractile ability and fluid builds up in your heart, it cannot efficiently pump blood, resulting in CHF, or congestive heart failure. Present in 2 percent of people ages 40 to 59 and 5 percent of those above 60, CHF reduces the degree of blood flow to your brain (hypoperfusion) and eventually results in dementia for a quarter of the people discharged from hospitals with this diagnosis.

Hypertension, or elevated blood pressure, raises your risk of stroke as well as congestive heart failure. Hypertension, just by itself, is highly associated with dementia. Dubbed a "silent killer" by the American Heart Association, hypertension is a condition with few apparent symptoms for many people. While having no symptoms might be seen as a positive feature, it often hides the problem and can fool you into believing you don't have it. As most people know, blood pressure is measured by taking a reading using a sphygmomanometer or blood pressure cuff. Over the last 50 years, our understanding of what constitutes a "good" blood pressure has evolved. Most recently, the National Institute of Aging and American Heart Association recommend keeping blood pressure at or below 120 mm HG systolic and 80 mm HG diastolic (120/80) for adults of all ages. The good news is that a meta-analysis of multiple well-controlled studies, published in 2020, found that treatment with antihypertensive (blood pressure lowering) medications significantly reduced the risk of new-onset dementia and cognitive impairment over the following four years.

# Type 2 Diabetes

Increasing evidence demonstrates that type 2 diabetes (T2DM) leads to significant likelihood of dementia. A 2016 study of over 1.5 million people found a 55 percent higher risk of dementia for people suffering from T2DM, the most common form of diabetes. This form of diabetes affects over 9 percent of the world's population, impacting some 460 million people between ages 20 and 79. Its incidence continues to rise with age, with a rate of 18 percent for those 65 years of age and older. T2DM arises from multiple genes interacting with a person's lifestyle and environment.

In the earliest stages, T2DM is marked by insulin resistance. Insulin is a hormone the body uses to move glucose, a sugar, from our blood into cells—especially brain cells—where it is converted into the energy molecule ATP. When the body cannot use the insulin correctly to get the glucose inside the cell, the glucose builds up outside the cells. This causes injury and damage to nerves, blood vessels, and organs throughout the body. Research has consistently shown that hyperglycemia, or a high glucose level, causes myocardial infarctions (MIs or heart attack) and worsens other heart abnormalities. It also leads to cardiovascular disease and the cerebrovascular events (CVAs and TIAs) that were discussed in the previous section. Hyperglycemia also causes neuropathy (nerve cell injury), nephropathy (chronic kidney disease), and retinopathy (irreversible damage to the retina of the eye that causes blindness). So, hyperglycemia is a starting point for a host of serious medical problems.

Insulin resistance is complicated. It reflects the interactions between our genes, in utero (during pregnancy) exposure to maternal high glucose levels, and early-life programming for energy metabolism. These factors are linked to and magnified when someone is overweight and physically inactive.

T2DM is most common in middle-aged and older adults, although it is increasingly being detected in children and adolescents. Its roots may appear during a pregnancy. If a woman develops gestational diabetes (GDM), she is twice as likely to develop T2DM in the 5 to 10 years after her pregnancy. And it is not just her health. Babies born to mothers with GDM are more likely to develop obesity as well as to double their rate of T2DM by age 22. So, the impact of diabetes begins at an early age and continues throughout our lives.

How do you know if you are developing diabetes? It comes down to a blood test. While short-term blood sugar levels are tested by fasting glucose levels (when they draw your blood before you have eaten that day), longer-term blood sugar control is better measured by Hemoglobin A1c (HbA1c). Your A1c level tells the doctor what the average blood sugar concentration has been for the last 90 days, the period of time when existing red blood cells are replaced by new ones. An A1c level below 5.7 percent is considered normal; 5.7–6.4 percent indicates insulin-resistance, a state that precedes outright diabetes and is often called "prediabetes." And, once it reaches 6.5 percent or higher, it is diagnosable as diabetes. Research published in 2013 examined the relationship between glucose levels and new cases of dementia in more than 2,000 people over five years. The findings were surprising. Even for people in the normal range of blood glucose levels, higher levels of glucose resulted in increased risk of dementia. Let's be clear: this relationship was found for people who were not yet diabetic. When you fall into the prediabetes range, your risk of dementia increases by 50 percent. And when your A1c rises to diabetic levels, your dementia risk doubles.

While you cannot change some of your diabetes risk factors— genetics, age, or ethnicity—you can modify your risk for developing it by making dietary changes and increasing your physical activity. TD2M is also treated successfully by medications that impact insulin resistance and blood sugar levels. In one study, newly diagnosed diabetes patients who were treated with oral medicines had a significant decrease in their dementia risk. This finding was echoed by a later study of over 170,000 people with diabetes who were followed for 17 years: controlling hyperglycemia and hyperinsulinemia significantly reduced their dementia risk.

Because both hypertension and T2DM are successfully treated by medications that are commonly available and relatively inexpensive, it is important for anyone with these conditions to take their medications every day, as directed by their doctor. Because many people in midlife with T2DM and hypertension lead very busy lives and all of us have less-than-perfect memory abilities, you may benefit from using a weekly pill container with separate compartments for each dosing time of the day. If you take a number of medications and have a complicated dosing schedule, you might benefit from an automatic pill dispenser that you have to prefill as infrequently as once a month. Such dispensers, either purchased or available through monthly subscription leasing programs, will deliver exactly the pills you need when you need them, remind you with a sound alarm, and even send you a message to your cell phone if you miss a dose. Because missing medication doses for either hypertension or diabetes may not have immediately noticeable consequences, you will not have an internal signal that tells you that you missed your medication that day. Technology could be your answer.

## Obesity

Obesity plays a significant role in vascular health, both directly and indirectly. Obesity is typically measured as body mass index, or BMI, the relationship between your weight and your height. While this is not a perfect measure, since it may miscalculate obesity in someone with a lot of muscle mass or particularly heavy bones, it is still a valuable general measure of your weight in relation to your height.

A "normal" BMI is 18.5–24.9 and is referred to as an "ideal" body weight. A BMI between 25 and 29.9 is considered overweight. BMIs over 30 fall into three classes of obesity. A BMI of 30 to 35 is Class 1, from 35 to under 40 represents Class 2, and a BMI of 40 or above, called Class 3 obesity, is severe.

You can calculate your BMI by using the online calculator offered by the National Institutes of Health at https://www.nhlbi.nih.gov/health /educational/lose_wt/BMI/bmicalc.htm. All you need to know is your height and weight.

Obesity is a very serious health problem in America. The most recent research finds that 40 percent of Americans are now classified as obese or very obese. By the year 2030, half of all Americans are projected to fall into the obese category, with 25 percent of us becoming classified as very obese. Please understand that this is not a moral judgment. We are not attempting to shame anyone or add to their psychological burden. Most people do not set out to become overweight and often have tried diligently not to become obese. But the facts tell us that weighing too much for our size is simply not good for our health and particularly for our brains. Obesity is a major driver of dementia risk and needs to be addressed in any approach to improving your brain health.

Moreover, obesity rarely occurs in isolation. When obesity is combined with high blood pressure, insulin resistance, and elevated LDL cholesterol or high triglycerides, the combination creates a "perfect storm" of health-challenging factors known as metabolic syndrome. The combination of these raises your risk of dying younger and increases your risk of dementia beyond the individual risk from any of these conditions alone.

The challenge of obesity lies in how to reduce its occurrence. Clearly, it does not begin overnight or arrive suddenly to someone who has otherwise had normal BMI, unless there is some other acute medical condition. Instead, it begins prenatally, in childhood, or in early to middle adulthood. It is impacted by a variety of medical conditions, socioeconomic factors, access to healthy diet options, race, and cultural programming. Obesity results from metabolic disturbance, dietary choices and habits, depression, unhealthy relationships with food, and sedentary lifestyle. As a result, the obesity epidemic in developed countries fuels the dementia epidemic of the future.

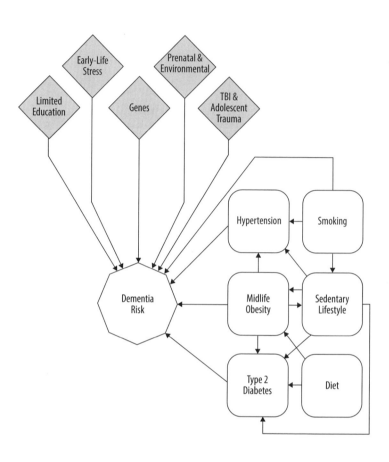

## CHAPTER 5

# Lifestyle Factors of Smoking, Diet, and Exercise

Hypertension and cardiovascular illness, midlife obesity, insulin resistance and type 2 diabetes, and elevated LDL cholesterol and triglyceride levels don't occur in a vacuum. Behind these accelerators of dementia risk there are lifestyle factors—smoking, poor diet, and physical inactivity—that create or worsen those medical conditions.

## Smoking Tobacco

Smoking cigarettes is clearly bad for your health, causing half a million deaths in the United States each year. To put that in perspective, it is the equivalent of all deaths due to HIV, illegal drug use, alcohol use, traffic accidents, and firearms *combined*. Cigarettes are responsible for 90 percent of lung cancers and 80 percent of chronic obstructive pulmonary disease (COPD), which is also life-threatening. You should also know that the effects of nicotine and carbon monoxide in cigarette smoke reduce the amount of oxygen reaching your heart and brain. They damage the lining of your blood vessels and cause atherosclerotic plaques, which eventually rupture, doubling to quadrupling your risk of heart attacks and strokes. To make matters worse, in smokers who also have hypertension, hypercholesterolemia, glucose intolerance, or diabetes, there is an interaction effect: cigarettes magnify these negative health consequences.

And, as you may imagine, these problems do not exclude your brain. Smoking, combined with other cardiovascular effects, causes brain atrophy, or shrinkage, which can be measured on an MRI. In a study looking at the MRI data from over 17,000 people, brain cell loss in smokers was much worse than that in nonsmokers. And this atrophy results in reduced cognitive ability. In other words, the brain of a smoker looks and acts "older" than that which is typical for that person's chronological age. The bottom line is that tobacco abuse is one of the most preventable causes of dementia.

## Diet

"What should I eat to prevent dementia?" is a common question that we encounter. We, as Americans, are obsessed with eating our way to better health and, as well, to dementia prevention. Dark-green vegetables, blue or purple fruits, chocolate, fish and chicken instead of beef, high fiber, low carb, low fat, vegan, vegetarian, Keto, you name it. You can buy books about eating an Alzheimer's prevention diet. Adding to the "eat this, not that" approach, intermittent fasting proponents believe that what you eat is less important than when you eat. They espouse limiting yourself to certain hours or certain days, with fasting during the other times. While you can make a good case that there are a number of foods that will drive up your weight, increase your insulin resistance, and contribute to hypertension, there are no magical foods that are proven to reduce your risk simply by eating a lot of them. Even for foods (such as oatmeal) that have shown evidence of reducing cholesterol levels, the effects are modest and, by themselves, ineffective in someone with true hypercholesterolemia.

And then there are the dietary supplements. In the late 1990s, an influential paper suggested that the herb Gingko biloba was likely effective in preventing Alzheimer disease through an antioxidant mechanism. Despite failure to replicate these initially optimistic findings and a large-scale study in 2008 in which no benefit was found, it remains a popular and highly profitable nonprescription remedy, either alone or when combined with other ingredients. The more recent "oral fixation for dementia prevention" that populates the television advertising world was advanced by a company claiming that their protein product from glowing jellyfish "supported brain function, [a] sharper mind, and clearer thinking." Or at least it used to make this claim before a nationwide class action lawsuit resulted in negotiated financial damages for its more than 3 million customers and a change in its advertising strategy. These days you are more likely to see a "pharmacist" recommending it or testimonials from older people who say that they believe that it helped their brains to think better again. But to be clear, a testimonial is not evidence and we advise our patients against its use.

There are, and will be more, dementia prevention products available online and in pharmacies, but buyer beware! Talk to your doctor first. If there was a nonprescription additive or medication proven to truly prevent dementia, we and doctors like us would be recommending or prescribing it. We would not be the last to know. But the evidence is not there and, as you are learning, dementia is such a complex process that there is a low probability that any one "pill" will prevent cognitive loss.

There is little evidence that adding coconut oil, garlic, or turmeric to your food will make a difference in your dementia risk, although some evidence points to dietary changes that lower blood pressure and, indirectly, reduce dementia likelihood. The "heart-healthy" Mediterranean diet and a variant, called MIND (Mediterranean–DASH Intervention for Neurodegenerative Delay), emphasizes eating whole grains, fruits and vegetables, olive oil, poultry, fish, and legumes, while avoiding salt, eggs, sugar, and red meat. In a 2015 study of people ages 58 to 98, those who adhered closely to these dietary principles had reduced dementia risk over the ensuing four and a half years. Similarly, an analysis of 10 randomized controlled trials of varying durations, concentrating on a ketogenic approach (primarily emphasizing protein and fat and minimizing carbohydrates), demonstrated improvement in general cognition and episodic memory (story recall), although genetic (*APOE* $\epsilon$4) status factored into the results.

Before you purge your pantry of foods not on the MIND diet, take a look at the calorie levels of what you are eating. Many of the dietary questions are ultimately answered by weight. When you maintain your BMI between 18.5 and 24.9, you will reduce your risk of cardiovascular disease, your blood pressure, and your periods of hyperglycemia. You will most often have better cholesterol and less chance of developing obstructive sleep apnea and metabolic syndrome. In the final analysis, it often comes down to calories consumed and calories burned.

Calorie restriction may need to be part of your dementia prevention plan if you are overweight or obese. But that is not the whole story. While it is true that the calorie intake you need daily to maintain your current weight depends on your gender, age, and activity level, some part of your hunger and food cravings may be regulated by your gut hormones and circadian rhythms. These two elements may determine how often you think about eating, why you have seemingly insatiable cravings, and why some of us have much greater difficulty losing weight, regardless of how much we eat and how much we exercise.

The real issue goes all the way back to evolution. Human beings needed a way to survive through extended periods of diminished food supplies. The solution was elegant, back then. When excess food was available, you ate it, and the body converted it all to fat, literally. Then, when the hunting parties were less than successful or winter was upon you, your body could convert the fat back into the glucose it needed to keep the brain and the rest of the body alive.

Signals from the body to the brain about when, what, and how much to eat developed into the elegant, intricate communication network that we are just beginning to fully appreciate today. We are coming to understand that the disease of obesity is really a disease of "energy dysregulation." In other words, for some people, getting to a healthy weight may involve a new class of medications to reset your body's energy "fat mass set point." For some people, the answer involves correcting their resistance to leptin, a food-intake suppressing hormone that fat cells release. For others, it may involve regulating hormones that you secrete from your intestinal cells when you start to eat. If your release level is too low or your release rate is too slow, your brain may be thinking you are still hungry long after you are satisfied. That makes it pretty hard to put down the fork or stay away from a snack two hours after dinner.

Science is still trying to identify why some peoples' fat mass set point is messed up from childhood on. It may be genetic, it may be caused by your mother being overweight during your pregnancy, or it may be due to how your body responded to food during infancy and childhood. We know that about 20 percent of children in the United States are already overweight. We also know that our fat mass set point seems to shift upwards as we age, with about two out of three adults in the United States suffering from overweight or obesity. Because excess weight is linked to most major illnesses that you can develop (heart attack, cancer, diabetes) as well as dementia, there is an increasing emphasis on using anti-obesity drugs as well as bariatric surgery. From a dementia prevention perspective, some people will very likely need more than diet and exercise, the basic "calories in versus calories out" equation. They may need medications or even surgery to achieve a healthy weight.

So, to start, your caloric need can be found at https://health.gov /our-work/food-nutrition/2015-2020-dietary-guidelines/guidelines /appendix-2/. Estimates for people of all age ranges are included. An adult woman maintains her weight with fewer calories than a man. If she is sedentary and not specifically exercising, consuming about 1,600 calories per day will keep her weight from changing. If she has an active lifestyle, such as walking more than three miles per day at three to four miles per hour, she may burn up to 2,400 calories daily. By comparison, a sedentary man's break-even point is 2,000 calories a day compared with an active man who burns about 3,000 calories daily. Another factor is age. Our metabolic rate slows down as we get older, so we will gain weight at age 50 by consuming the same level of calories that we did when we were 30. Not a surprise for most of us, as we think back to the glory days of our youth when we could stuff ourselves without letting out the waistband in our pants.

Notice that these recommendations take into account the amount and degree of physical activity. Ultimately, whether you are at a body mass that is healthy for your brain and your heart, it boils down to calories: how many you take in versus how many you burn off. Despite our best attempts to circumvent a basic law of nature, if we consume more calories than we burn off on a daily basis, our body stores the extra calories in the form of body fat. Those excess calories, regardless of whether they come from carbohydrates, proteins, or fats, will be stored as body fat. And the research demonstrates that the fatter we are around our middle, the thinner we are in the surface of our brains.

## Exercise and Sedentary Lifestyle

Physical exercise has long been accepted as part of a comprehensive treatment plan for people with cardiac conditions, lung disease, diabetes, and elevated cholesterol. More recent data underscore the importance of exercise for brain activity by focusing on the underlying mechanisms. Exercise increases the oxygen available to our cells, increases specific chemical and cellular factors important in cell growth and repair, and decreases cardio- and cerebrovascular risks. Exercise has been shown to improve attention focusing, reduce depression, and modulate the inflammatory processes seen in metabolic disorders. Consistent evidence demonstrates clear differences in the rates of dementia and the size of specific brain regions in people who exercise versus those who do not. One study estimated that consistent exercise essentially turns back the aging process by one to two years.

But you do not have to take up marathon or triathlon training. Even low to moderate activity levels protect against cognitive decline, with more vigorous levels conferring an even greater beneficial effect. Regular physical exercise increases the amount of gray matter in the brain while sedentary behavior, just doing what someone needs to do to get through an average day, results in more brain shrinkage. And the research demonstrates that whether the exercise is aerobic or resistance training, it doesn't matter, as both are proven to delay cognitive decline.

The Physical Activity Guidelines for Americans 2015–2020 suggests that a minimum daily exercise regimen for people 18 to 64 years old should include at least 150 minutes a week of moderate-intensity or 75 minutes of vigorous-intensity aerobic physical activity. The guidelines also note that someone who wants the maximal health benefit should double those amounts.

Not surprisingly, cardiorespiratory fitness (CRF), a measure of physical activity, throughout one's lifetime is related to cognition in later life, with better CRF in early adulthood pointing to better memory and processing speed in midlife. Even individuals in their 70s demonstrated that an increased number of steps they took while walking, and the increased heart rate that went with it, improved their overall cognition. Importantly, even for individuals who are already demonstrating cognitive loss, numerous studies show that exercise slows cognitive decline. That is why we, along with the American Academy of Neurology, recommend that all of our patients exercise regularly, regardless of their current level of cognition.

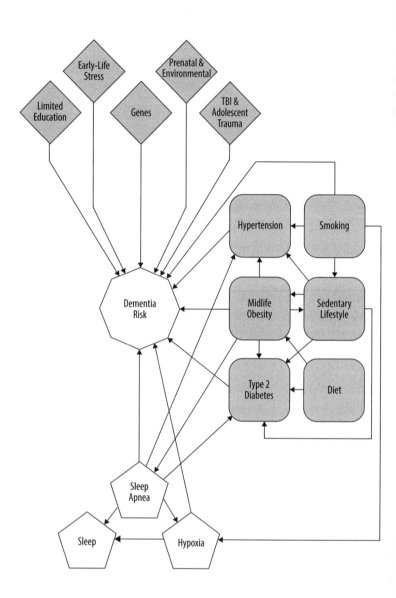

## CHAPTER 6

# Sleeping, Breathing, Breathing while Sleeping

## The Importance of Sleep

You likely have had a few bad nights of sleep throughout your life. You have difficulty falling asleep or you wake up and can't get back to sleep. You may be anxious about an upcoming problem, worried about your health, depressed about a loss, or excited about tomorrow's trip. Or maybe your teething 2-year-old crawled into bed with you, your back is in pain, you drank a few too many beers, or you are pregnant. You are not alone. One in three Americans, according to the Centers for Disease Control and Prevention (CDC), report that they do not get enough sleep. And, one in a hundred, according to recent data, suffers from chronic insomnia, such that they spend most or all nights struggling to get enough hours of uninterrupted sleep. Sleep disruption becomes very common in older adults, where 50 percent report at least one problem with sleep most nights.

How much sleep is enough? We used to believe that everyone needed a solid eight hours every night. More recently, six to eight hours is thought to be the best for most people, with adolescents needing more and older adults possibly needing less.

While busy and hard-working people view sleep as wasted time, we now understand that sleep is important for health. Valuable metabolic, emotional, and cognitive functions occur while we sleep, and insufficient amounts of sleep are linked to a number of medical conditions, including hypertension, diabetes, obesity, heart attack, stroke, depression, and automobile accidents. Many medical residency programs now place greater limits on the shift lengths that young doctors can work to reduce medical errors. In the transportation industry, both truck drivers and airline personnel are limited in their hours of work to improve alertness and safety.

Even in young, healthy adults, research has shown decreases in reaction time and vigilance on cognitive testing after only a few days of modest (4–6 hours) sleep restriction.

So, what about dementia? Sleep and dementia risk is an evolving area of interest, with much of the research occurring in the last five years. Reviews of the literature published in 2017 and 2018 found 50 percent higher rates for dementia and all-cause mortality in older people with sleep fragmentation. A 2019 study showed that sleep disturbances and abnormal sleep duration were associated with Alzheimer disease likelihood as well as its progression. Conversely, older adults who report getting good sleep and feeling refreshed when they awake show better thinking. As we will see later, when obstructive sleep apnea is part of the problem, there is an even stronger link between disrupted sleep and impaired thinking.

Most recently, a 2021 analysis of 2,800+ older adults over a five-year period in the United States discovered that those who slept five or fewer hours per night had more than twice the risk of dementia and twice the risk of death.

While you know that you are not at your best after a poor night's sleep, the effects of more chronic sleep impairment may be harder to appreciate. You can become numb to your sleep deprivation and

often develop bad sleep habits, such as compensatory daytime napping, going to bed very early and watching TV or reading until you fall
asleep, or surfing the Internet and playing games on your cell phone or
tablet without realizing that blue light emissions are waking up your
brain. You may have begun to rely on nonprescription sleep aids, marijuana, and some prescription drugs to temporarily overcome your
insomnia. After a while you have muddled the normal sleep patterns
to such an extent that you have lost your normal patterns or stages of
healthy sleep. But the mechanism for how this could lead to dementia
is only very recently becoming understood.

The first thing to remember is that your brain is working all the
time, even when you are asleep. Learning new information and building new connections between neurons takes lots of raw materials,
work, and energy. And, just like most manufacturing plants, the process also creates waste products. In the brain, some of the waste molecules, like tau protein and beta-amyloid, are toxic to brain cells, even in
minute amounts.

This is where sleep comes in: the glymphatic system, or the waste
removal system in the brain, is most active during the deeper stage of
sleep, or non-REM sleep as opposed to REM, or rapid eye movement
sleep, when dreaming occurs. So, non-REM sleep is where your brain
is flushing away the still soluble forms of these cellular poisons before
they can kill neurons (nerve cells) and glia (support cells). In 2018, scientists showed that even one night of sleep deprivation increased the
amount of soluble beta-amyloid in the brain of a healthy person, irrespective of their *APOE* €4 risk for Alzheimer disease.

So, whether your sleep architecture is repeatedly disrupted by a
newborn's two-hour feeding schedule, job-shift changes, pain, staying
up to get extra work or studying done, or the hypoxia of sleep apnea,
when you alter the number of hours and type of sleep you get, you
are hampering your brain's ability to clear away garbage. There is not

enough nightly custodial service in your brain's "office" to empty the trash cans and clean off the surfaces. Not surprisingly, scientists have also found that many conditions associated with all-cause dementia, such as obesity, lack of exercise, hypertension, insulin resistance and diabetes, cerebral infarction (strokes/TIAs) and brain bleeds, as well as clogged blood vessels in the brain (cerebral atherosclerosis) are all associated with dysfunction in the brain's glymphatic system. This new data about our "sleeping" brain promises new avenues for even earlier interventions for dementia prevention in the coming years.

## The Importance of Breathing

Habitually late, Dr. Peter Safar, the guest speaker at the 1961 commencement of the University of Pittsburgh Medical School and the father of CPR (cardiopulmonary resuscitation), entered the majestic Carnegie Music Hall from the rear, strode down the long center aisle, past the audience, and up to the stage. After he was introduced, he stood quietly, gazing out at the large assembly of new doctors, their families, and faculty. Then, he stated, "Pink is good. Blue is bad. Air must go in and out. And that's all you need to know." Without another word, Dr. Safar left the stage and a stunned audience.

Dr. Safar's admonition remains as true today as it was 60 years ago. Oxygen is essential for life, and particularly for thinking. Getting that oxygen out of the air, into your blood, and out to all the parts of your body, especially your brain, is central for dementia prevention.

Why is oxygen so important? Because your cells require oxygen in order to make energy molecules called ATP (adenosine triphosphate). Insufficient oxygen reduces or eliminates ATP, causing your cells to stop working and eventually die. And this oxygen has to be present constantly. Depending on your individual metabolic rate, you only have enough oxygen in your blood to last up to three to four minutes. Hypoxia, or oxygen deprivation, for longer periods can cause irreversible cerebral damage or death. But, as we now know, hypoxia doesn't have to be a single event. Repeated episodes of milder, intermittent hypoxia persisting over time will cause major changes in brain cell and molecular functions. Ultimately, such changes interfere with effective thinking.

The complex brain activities involved in thinking—paying attention, making decisions, remembering, communicating—require a network of 100 billion neurons and an almost equal number of glial support cells. All of these cells require an uninterrupted, 24-hour supply of energy. And energy requires oxygen.

So, the bottom line is simple: we have to breathe, at a rate of 12 to 20 breaths per minute in order to get enough oxygen to remain alive. And, we have to do this even when we're sleeping.

Here is where it gets a little technical. Oxygen makes up only 20 percent of the air you breathe (the rest is mostly nitrogen). It must first get down to your lungs so that it can be absorbed into your bloodstream through structures called alveoli. Oxygen molecules then "hook up" or bind to red blood cells that carry iron-containing hemoglobin (iron makes them red in color) to every part of your body, especially to your brain where it is used to make the ATP energy molecules. Carbon dioxide is a by-product of the cellular energy manufacturing process, so for every breath of air you inhale, you need to exhale carbon dioxide. As Dr. Safar said, "Air must go in and out."

The amount of oxygen in the air you breathe is also important, as hemoglobin in the red blood cells can only capture whatever amount of oxygen is available in the lungs. If you are a healthy adult, you need to maintain a 95 percent or greater oxygen saturation level in your blood to ensure that your neurons work properly. When your blood is "well saturated" you will typically have pink lips and nailbeds. As Dr. Safar noted, "Pink is good."

But other factors can affect how much oxygen is in the air, including high altitude. This can become a problem in certain geographic locations, but it is a particular problem for someone flying at more than 10,000 feet without oxygen supplementation. Early military experiments in the late 1930s found that pilots flying above that level became inattentive, mentally inefficient, emotionally variable, depressed, and irritable. They had reduced hearing and vision. Surprisingly, they were generally unaware that anything was wrong! They thought they had performed splendidly.

It turns out that you don't have to fly above 10,000 feet to suffer from hypoxia and to experience problems with thinking and emotion. These same cognitive changes will occur in anyone who has too little oxygen for their red blood cells to transport to their brain. In this state of oxygen "desaturation," when levels fall at or below 90 percent, their lips and nailbeds become cyanotic or turn blue. Again, as Dr. Safar noted, "Blue is bad." Low levels of oxygen, or hypoxia, can occur as a result of pulmonary problems, such as chronic obstructive pulmonary disease (COPD), a result of cigarette smoking, asbestos exposure, air pollution, some pneumonias, and genetics. Whatever the cause, too little oxygen increases the risk for cognitive problems.

## The Importance of Breathing While You Sleep: Sleep Apnea

So here is where we put it together. For many people who later develop cognitive problems, they do not get enough air to their lungs while they sleep, so not enough oxygen can be pulled from the air and can make its way to their brain. This condition is called sleep apnea. Sleep apnea is the most common type of sleep-disordered breathing (SDB), estimated to affect one in four middle-aged adults in the United States. Despite this very high prevalence, only 10 percent of the population has been adequately screened and only 20 percent are diagnosed.

Normally, as you breathe, air goes to the back of your throat, down your airway or "windpipe," and into your lungs. Not all airways are the same size. Some people are born with smaller airways and others are crowded by their tonsils and adenoids, by the size of their tongue, or by their uvula, that tissue hanging in the back of your throat that looks somewhat like a punching bag. These structures do not pose much of a problem when you're awake because your brain automatically compensates by increasing the activity of the muscles that keep your airway open.

But things change when you sleep, especially in the stage when you dream. During this dream period, called REM, or rapid eye movement, your airway muscles relax, just like all the rest of the muscles in your body to keep you from acting out dreams. Unfortunately, in people with obstructive sleep apnea (OSA), these muscles become too relaxed and the airway collapses. Despite your struggle to breathe, the net result is that not enough air gets to your lungs and not enough oxygen can get pulled from your lungs and into your bloodstream. Not enough air, not enough oxygen to your brain.

A few technical terms for you. *Apnea* refers to a pause in respiration for at least 10 seconds even though you are still trying to take a breath. *Hypopnea* is a partial or incomplete interruption of breathing where your oxygen level drops by at least 4 percent for 10 seconds. The diagram in figure 6.1 shows these structures and contrasts normal breathing with apneas.

In "obstructive" sleep apnea, your airway is blocked or collapses. In "central" sleep apnea, on the other hand, your brain fails to signal your body to take a breath. The causes of central apnea are more complex but reflect factors that are "central" to how your brain regulates and controls your breathing efforts. People who suffer from both types of apneas are diagnosed with complex sleep apnea.

So how do you know if you have sleep apnea? While there are some common symptoms, including daytime fatigue, early evening dozing, snoring, gasping for air, awakening repeatedly to urinate, waking up with headaches, and feeling exhausted in the morning, the only true way to diagnose sleep apnea is with an overnight sleep test. We know, you always wanted to sleep through a test. But, in this case, whether the test is a home sleep study (HST) or a test conducted in a sleep lab, called a polysomnogram (PSG), you are connected to telemetry devices that continuously measure your heart rate, respiration or breathing rate, oxygen level, and the number of your arousals from sleep and leg movements. If you have this test in a lab, your brain waves (EEG) are also typically recorded.

A number of different scores are calculated from a sleep study, but the one most often used diagnostically is the apnea-hypopnea index (AHI). This combines the number of times you stop breathing (apneas)

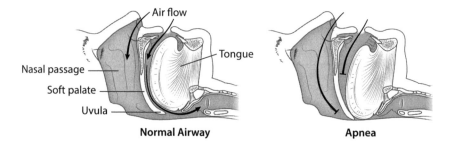

**Normal Airway**     **Apnea**

FIGURE 6.1. A normal airway contrasted with a complete airway obstruction resulting in apnea. SOURCE: Adapted from Hahn PY, Somers VK. Sleep apnea and hypertension. In: Lip GYH, Hall JE, eds. *Comprehensive Hypertension*. St. Louis, MO: Mosby; 2007:201–207. Used with permission from Elsevier.

with the number of times your oxygen level drops (hypopneas) and divides this by the number of hours you slept—sort of like miles per gallon calculation for cars. The in-lab PSG can also give important data regarding oxygen levels at different stages of sleep and sleeping position as well as heart rate. It can also differentiate between obstructive and central apneas.

The standard rule for adults is that an AHI of 5.0 or more (breath stoppages plus oxygen drops per hour) leads to a diagnosis of apnea. An AHI of 5–15 is considered mild, 16–30 is moderate, and 31 or more indicates severe apnea. But you should not confuse mild OSA with insignificant OSA. Even mild apnea is a significant problem. Losing oxygen five or more times per hour makes an impact on your brain and has negative effects on your cardiovascular and metabolic health as well as your quality of life.

Mild but significant sleep apnea was the case for Jimmie. Jimmie thought that his sleep patterns were "pretty normal for a guy in his 50s." He had the "normal" waking up at 2:00 a.m. and 4:00 a.m. to use the bathroom, the "normal" falling asleep during the later innings of the baseball game, and the "normal" snoring (which he thought his wife was making up just to get his goat). He had already had a sleep study, about three years ago, which he told us was "normal, just mild apnea." He was shocked when we told him that mild sleep apnea meant that he "only" stopped breathing 5 to 15 times every hour while he slept. He was even more surprised when we explained that some of his word-finding problems, forgetting to turn off the stove burner, and repeatedly losing his car keys in the house could be caused by his brain's lack of oxygen. Not to mention the half-hour naps he was sneaking at his desk to recharge his batteries and make it through the work day.

Mild sleep apnea is not insignificant sleep apnea, and it certainly is not normal sleep. Ideally, you should be breathing whenever you are sleeping, with only an occasional episode of reduced oxygen.

## *Sleep Apnea and Cognitive Decline*

With too little oxygen making its way through the circulatory system to the brain, particularly over extended periods of time, neurons are altered, injured, or killed. This damage interferes with brain function and creates problems with your ability to think.

When the oxygen loss is minimal, no one, including the person who is affected, may notice. But, as oxygen deficits persist or worsen, you and those around you may start to notice something being slightly off in your thinking or behavior. You are more easily distracted, struggle to find words, forget your intentions, act somewhat differently, and make careless mistakes. These are especially noticeable if you are stressed, tired, or ill, such as with an infection. These prolonged hypoxic injuries to your neurons or to the connections in your neuronal network may have led to mild cognitive impairment (MCI). In MCI, sensitive cognitive tests show a decline in one or more critical areas of your thinking but your everyday functions are still generally preserved.

However, when hypoxia injures enough neurons and disrupts enough of the brain's networks, more profound changes in thinking occur and interfere with a person's everyday function. By then, MCI has likely progressed into dementia. Clear impairment can now usually be found in two areas of cognition, such as language, decision-making, orientation and visual spatial relations, as well as memory.

The connection between medical conditions that produced hypoxia and cognitive problems was observed in the mid-1980s by specialists in pulmonology, cardiology, neurology, psychiatry, and internal medicine, although these were largely separate observations. It didn't matter if it was pneumonia that prevented oxygen exchange with carbon dioxide in the alveoli of the lungs or whether the patient's air sacs were destroyed by lung cancer or COPD, dementia occurred at far higher than expected rates. It didn't matter if blood was blocked from getting to the brain by a clot during an ischemic stroke or if heart muscle failure of disrupted heart rhythms caused the drop in blood flow, the outcome was often irreparable cognitive loss.

Around the same time, other researchers examined dementia patients who were thought to have Alzheimer disease based on the diagnostic criteria in the 1980s and found they had a 10-fold higher rate of obstructive sleep apnea when compared to people who weren't experiencing dementia. Thirty years later, in 2016, when slightly more rigorous criteria were used for the clinical diagnosis of Alzheimer disease, a large meta-analysis (a statistical review combining data from smaller studies) found that individuals with Alzheimer disease had five times the rate of sleep-disordered breathing than people without dementia.

Additional links between hypoxia-related medical conditions and dementia were subsequently found in patients with COPD in 1993, in stroke patients in 1994, and in congestive heart disease patients in 1996. By 2007, hypoxia caused by blood flow changes (hypoxic ischemia) from traumatic brain injury were linked with later dementia. In 2011, acute oxygen deprivation after a heart attack or cardiac arrest was shown to cause an immediate upsurge in beta-amyloid production in the brain, the same beta-amyloid that Alois Alzheimer reported as a hallmark of dementia in 1906.

It is now generally accepted that hypoxia precipitates a biochemical cascade of widespread injury throughout the body, increasing blood pressure, altering heart rate, abnormally triggering stress hormones and inflammatory responses, impairing metabolic regulation and blood flow, and interfering with the production of neurotransmitters, the proteins and chemicals we need for healthy brain function. Not surprisingly, then, sleep apnea is causally linked to conditions known to be directly or indirectly related to dementia.

Sleep apnea is connected to coronary heart disease and heart attacks, abnormal heart rhythms like atrial fibrillation, congestive heart failure, hypertension, obesity, and diabetes. It also elevates your risk of stroke (CVA) and transient ischemic attacks (TIAs). Apnea is also linked to depression and anxiety. The hypoxia associated with sleep apnea also increases loss of kidney function and even causes erectile dysfunction. The net of it is this: sleep apnea, either directly or indirectly, triggers a host of medical problems, many of which increase the likelihood of developing dementia.

The second way in which sleep-disordered breathing impacts your thinking is through its fragmenting effect on your sleep. As you saw in the beginning of this chapter, sleep duration is important for your brain. But so is sleep continuity. There are specific sequences and stages of sleep that keep your physiological processes stable and that are necessary for normal thinking when you are awake.

Sleep-disordered breathing and sleep fragmentation caused by arousals as you attempt to breathe increase hyperactivity, irritability, impulsivity, and inattention, all characteristics of attention-deficit/hyperactivity disorder (ADHD). Twenty-five years of research has consistently demonstrated a relationship between sleep-disordered breathing and ADHD in children. In fact, a 1997 study by doctors at the University of Michigan suggested that the ADHD symptoms in 81 percent of children would be eliminated by treating their SDB.

The underlying mechanism involves the endothelium, the microscopic blood vessels that make up the blood–brain barrier (BBB), where oxygen is exchanged between the bloodstream and the brain. The BBB becomes disrupted in children with sleep apnea due to intermittent hypoxia and predicts cognitive deficits in 80 percent of the children.

Currently, the major treatment for children is surgical removal of their tonsils and adenoids. In children with mild apnea and ADHD, surgery improves attention, impulse control, and response time, although it is often not enough for older, obese, asthmatic, or more severely apneic children. Another approach, using continuous positive airway pressure (CPAP), has been shown in one early study in 2012 to restore memory functions and motor speed to normal.

ADHD is not just a childhood disorder. About half of children with ADHD continue to show this condition as adults. Here as well, adult ADHD is related to OSA: a 2019 study found that 83 percent of middle-aged adults who screened positive for ADHD had OSA, of which 60 percent of the cases were moderate or severe.

So, if you have children who have ADHD, you should be interested in knowing how they breathe while they sleep. Identifying and treating sleep apnea could prevent years of poor school performance, behavioral problems, and cognitive difficulty. They could go farther in school, which we know is protective against later cognitive decline. They will also be less impulsive and vulnerable to making bad decisions that are also related to later-life cognitive problems, including accidental head injury, binge drinking, and drug abuse. This OSA–ADHD connection was found in a 2011 study in which people with ADHD symptoms in early adulthood were five times more likely to develop dementia, specifically Lewy Body dementia (DLB), when they got older.

One of the myths about OSA is that it is mostly a man's disease, and particularly obese men with thick necks. Statistics show that men are diagnosed twice as frequently as women, but this is likely due to the under-diagnosis of women. One large study found that over 90 percent of women with moderate to severe OSA had not been diagnosed despite adequate access to medical care. Better data indicate that equal numbers of men and women have OSA by the time they reach their 50s.

How common is OSA in adults? The often-reported 1993 US statistic of 25 percent of men and 10 percent of women is likely an underestimate today, as our population is now older and more obese. OSA increases with age and is five times more common if you are over age 60 than if you are 25. In some cohorts older than 60, a 2017 research review reported OSA rates of 90 percent in men and nearly 80 percent in women! About half of these people had moderate levels. And while 75 percent of people with OSA have a body mass index (BMI) in the obese range, you do not have to be overweight. Some of our patients with moderate or severe apnea have been fashion-model thin.

How does SDB affect our cognition? At the most basic level it causes us to lose brain cells and the critical connectivity between brain cells that is the very foundation of thinking. Recent advanced neuroimaging has allowed us to see that people with OSA have a loss of neurons in regions sensitive to lack of oxygen, including the frontal, temporal, and parietal lobes of the brain and the cerebellum, as well as decreased size of the hippocampus, a central memory structure. These tests also showed "white matter hyperintensities" on MRI scans, a common result of small blood vessel changes found in vascular dementia. Biomarkers used to detect Alzheimer disease were similarly affected in middle-aged, cognitively normal individuals with untreated apnea.

In the last decade, more than 150 studies have examined the impact of sleep-disordered breathing on cognition. While there are differences in the specific findings among these studies, largely based on how they were constructed and the severity of OSA, the abundance of data indicates that adults with sleep apnea perform significantly worse than people of the same age on tests of attention, memory, problem-solving, processing speed, and other mental abilities. When brain cell and network activity are measured, we see that their brains actually have to work harder just to stay on par when performing a simple memory task. And while experts may disagree on all the steps in the causal pathway between OSA and dementia, the overwhelming evidence is that OSA, and the level of hypoxia that it causes, creates cognitive problems in middle-aged and elderly people and that those problems begin at an earlier age. The largest systematic analysis of such data, a 2017 analysis of more than 4 million mostly middle-aged people, revealed that people with sleep-disordered breathing already had worse executive function at baseline and were at 35 percent higher risk for developing cognitive impairment than other individuals. To put the risk in terms of time, researchers evaluating the Alzheimer's Disease Neuroimaging Initiative (ADNI) participants found that those with OSA experienced the onset of MCI and dementia 10 years earlier than those without it.

But what you also need to know is that OSA is more than a problem that can lead to serious medical conditions and a decline of brain function into mild cognitive impairment and dementia; it is also a treatable condition that offers a pathway to dementia prevention.

## The Importance of Treating Sleep Apnea

The primary treatment for OSA is continuous positive airway pressure (CPAP), a sophisticated, nonsurgical, non-pharmacological treatment that can improve or even normalize objectively measured cognitive losses. CPAP treatment can improve concentration, problem-solving, and short-term memory. Even just several weeks of CPAP treatment for Alzheimer's patients with OSA have demonstrated improved thinking while sustained CPAP use for 13 months has resulted in significantly less deterioration in global cognition compared with those who stopped using CPAP. The ADNI cohort study also found that CPAP use delayed the age when people developed mild cognitive impairment. And for the 40 to 60 percent of Parkinson disease patients who also have OSA, as little as three and a half hours of nightly CPAP use over 13 months showed improved cognition and reduced anxiety.

We also see positive changes on neuroimaging scans, with improved white matter after three months of CPAP use and nearly complete reversal of abnormalities after one year. Other studies demonstrate reduced thinning of the brain surface or cortex, improved neural network connectivity, and increased gray matter volume (number of cell bodies of neurons) in structures such as the hippocampus and thalamus, and in the frontal regions of the brain. Using CPAP for at least four hours per night over three months normalized brain activation areas and workload during memory testing of middle-aged patients with severe OSA. And, the pathological levels of Alzheimer's biomarkers found in the blood and cerebrospinal fluid of untreated OSA sufferers regained normal levels in those treated with CPAP.

This relationship between sleep-disordered breathing and cognition is what we call the "Brain–Breathing Connection." Such consistent findings suggest that we need to consider breathing and oxygen in any study of new medicines for dementia. They also suggest that we must identify and treat sleep apnea when it is present when someone comes into a doctor's office complaining of problems thinking or remembering. Of all the takeaways from this book, the Brain–Breathing Connection may be the most important.

## Signs and Symptoms of Obstructive Sleep Apnea

By now you may be wondering if you have obstructive sleep apnea. We have already touched on some symptoms that could prompt you to get an overnight sleep test. But just to summarize, here are the common ones:

- Snoring is common in 94 percent of people later diagnosed with sleep apnea. But, since many people without snoring never get a sleep study, not everyone with sleep apnea snores. Snoring is the wood-sawing sound you make when your airway is too small or begins to collapse. During snoring, when you struggle to breathe you have "micro-awakenings" in which you arouse from a deeper stage of sleep to a more alert level so your airway can open. Since you are still asleep when you snore, you may not even know that you do it. You may believe that your partner is complaining for no reason, and you may argue that you sleep "just fine." It may take your partner's cell phone recording of last night's sleep to bring home the message.

- *Nocturia* is the medical term for one or more episodes of urination at night. This symptom is not something that would spring to mind as being obviously connected to whether your brain has enough oxygen. While frequent nocturia is a hallmark of OSA, it is commonly misattributed to prostate problems in men and weakened bladder suspensory muscles in women. But, regardless of whether you drink water before going to sleep or not, the real mechanism involves hypoxia.

- At some point in the middle of the night, you are not breathing normally. Your brain becomes starved for oxygen, and messages the heart to "Send me more (oxygen rich) blood!" As you struggle to get air down your airway, and your brain is rousing you from a deep sleep, your heart is beating faster and pumping harder to get that blood up to the brain. All that stressful pumping of extra blood stretches the upper walls of the heart, mimicking congestive heart failure. This really gets your body's attention to reduce the fluid "overload." A hormone, ANP (atrial natriuretic peptide), released in the heart quickly signals your kidneys to make more urine, because this is the fastest way to get rid of excess blood volume. Your kidneys then make more urine, which fills up your bladder and wakes you up to urinate. But the strange thing is, one to two hours later, you have to go again, even though you did not drink anything. For those with apnea who do this repeatedly, we tell them, "It is not your prostate, it is not your bladder, it is your apnea."

- Recurrent headaches, especially in the morning, are also fairly common, linked to a buildup of carbon dioxide ($CO_2$) overnight combined with oxygen deficiency. Paradoxically, this may occur mostly on weekends when you sleep in. While you get more sleep, you spend more time getting less oxygen.

- A sore throat, hoarse voice, or dry tongue when you first wake up can be due to "mouth breathing," an unconscious and unsuccessful attempt to get more air down your trachea.

- Nonrestorative sleep is also common. You wake up feeling tired, even though you think you've slept eight hours, and you want more sleep just to get more energy. It may take several cups of coffee or tea just to get going. And you feel as if you are thinking through mud. You struggle to juggle several thoughts at once and your creativity is dampened. You feel yourself nodding and drifting off while reading or watching TV. You also need to make sure that you stay awake while waiting at the traffic light. In some cases, you may have wandered over the highway's center line because your brain just "went to sleep" with your eyes open, a series of millisecond "micronaps" while you need to be awake. Incidentally, alcoholic beverage or drug use makes us even more susceptible to these micronaps.

Let's look at the Brain–Breathing Connection for one of our patients.

# Charlie P.: A Case of Apparently Reversed Dementia

Charlie was distressed. At 57, this Vietnam vet was suffering from anxiety, insomnia, PTSD (posttraumatic stress disorder), and depression. He no longer enjoyed his hobbies, was distractible, and started forgetting simple facts and procedures he used to know. His slightly older wife was even more upset: Charlie was now having trouble keeping up with her.

He came to see us in 2007. His cognitive testing confirmed that he had significant weakness on tests of attention, problem-solving, and short-term memory. These were serious enough to be considered mild cognitive impairment or mild vascular dementia. Several months later, both an MRI (magnetic resonance imaging) and a PET (positron emission tomography) scan showed problems. The PET was particularly interesting. This scan reflects brain metabolism and reflects what parts of the brain are "lighting up" with brain activity and which parts are not so bright or active. After Charlie received a mildly radioactive infusion of a glucose solution through a vein in his arm, his brain was scanned to see how his brain was using this sugary fuel. The PET scan produced pictures that, to Charlie, looked like a Doppler radar weather image. Except, as we explained, here the PET "storms" were good, reflecting increased brain activity and the quieter, darker areas reflected problems.

Unfortunately, Charlie's PET scan showed a lot of dark areas where there should have been more activity. The neuroradiologist who interpreted the PET said that he had "early changes consistent with Alzheimer's disease."

We sat down with Charlie and his wife to discuss all the findings of his cognitive testing, his scans, and his blood tests. All pointed to our diagnosis of mild dementia. But we also had a plan. We urged him to lose weight, to exercise, and consistently take his diabetes, blood pressure, and depression medications. Charlie was interested in memory-sparing medications but was not at all interested in having a sleep study.

He returned several times over the next several months. He stopped the memory drugs and didn't want to try any others. He remained depressed, unmotivated, tired, overweight, and had to use the bathroom several times at night. His wife saw him declining and was even more concerned. At her persuasive insistence, Charlie eventually agreed to get a sleep study. He had moderate obstructive sleep apnea, with an AHI over 15.

Charlie then started using CPAP or continuous positive airway pressure, the gold-standard treatment for apnea. His CPAP machine sucked in room air through a filter, pressurized the air, humidified it, and sent it gently and quietly out the other end through a soft, flexible plastic tube connected to a mask he wore over his nose while sleeping. The pressured air kept Charlie's airway open while he slept and allowed more air to flow into his lungs when he breathed. With better breathing, more oxygen got to his brain.

When Charlie started CPAP, we emphasized that he needed to use it every night, for at least four hours, and preferably whenever he slept, even during naps. We told him that he needed to take his CPAP on vacation as well. The central message was, "Whenever you sleep, you should breathe." Charlie agreed and surprisingly found that CPAP was okay. He was particularly pleased that he did not have more pills to try to remember to take. Shortly after he started CPAP he came for his previously scheduled cognitive retesting. There was no significant change in test scores, nor were there any changes on a second PET scan.

Charlie did not return for two years. During this time, he had no changes in his health or his medicines, but Charlie had been using his CPAP—every night, all night. He had a third PET scan that was reviewed by the same neuroradiologist as before. But this time, the doctor was shocked: Charlie's PET scan was now entirely normal. Formerly darkened areas of the brain lit up brightly with brain activity and the radiologist concluded that Charlie had "reversed to normal from Alzheimer's."

Charlie's wife brought him back to see us. She wanted an explanation for this. He was definitely better, but his primary care doctor (who had been seeing him in the interim) couldn't explain it. He also could not explain why Charlie's blood pressure was under control and he didn't need diabetes or cholesterol medications any more. His weight was down. And Charlie had more energy. He was back to enjoying his hobbies and doing more activities with his wife. He even took up writing poetry, something he always wanted to do but could never start. His wife was delighted and amazed, happily rediscovering "the guy that I married!"

And, consistent with his PET scan, Charlie's cognitive test scores improved back to normal levels for his age. We presented a poster of Charlie's case, complete with his three PET scans, at the Alzheimer's Association International Conference in Vancouver in 2012. Our poster was titled "A Case of Apparently Reversed Alzheimer's Disease." (You can see the poster and Charlie's PET scans on our website at www.brain doc.com.)

We have also gathered data from 353 patients with cognitive complaints that we saw between 2009 and 2010, and we found that 64 percent of them had abnormally low oxygen levels, either at rest, when walking, or sleeping at night. By 2014, our data on another 328 patients presented at the annual meeting of the American Academy of Neurology documented that 82 percent of these patients with cognitive complaints had hypoxia at rest, with ambulation, or while sleeping.

While Charlie's case is dramatic, it is entirely true and shares a glimpse of how hypoxia induced by sleep apnea can impact cognitive loss and how effective treatment may improve someone's thinking and even prevent dementia. Charlie's experience with breathing and thinking has been mirrored by hundreds of other patients in our practice. Pink is definitely good.

We last saw Charlie in 2019. At 12 years from his first appointment, now 69 years old, Charlie continues to do very well, has not developed dementia, and is on his third CPAP machine. We still have the signed first edition copy of his poetry book and the picture of the roses he brought in on the first anniversary of his last PET scan.

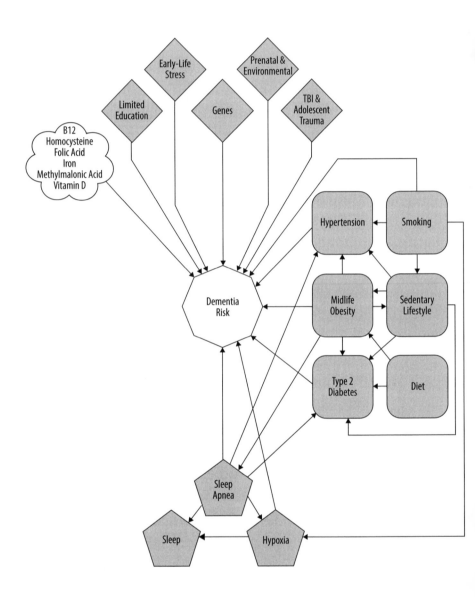

## CHAPTER 7

# Metabolic and Vitamin Deficiencies

Vitamins and herbal remedies are big business. A 2019 survey by a leading trade association, the Council for Responsible Nutrition (CRN), reported that 76 percent of Americans reported taking vitamins and minerals on a regular basis. According to the US Food and Drug Administration (FDA), supplements are a booming business. In 2019, the market exceeded 40 billion dollars.

It's a very long way from where it all started in 1912 when a Polish biochemist, Casimir Funk, published his first paper about "vital amines" or "life-giving amines," which he believed were needed, albeit in small amounts, for your body to work properly. His work sparked the subsequent discovery of 13 other vitamins in the next several decades.

Funk's original hypothesis was that a specific disease was caused by a specific deficiency in one of these nutrients and that replacing the "vital amine" would cure the disease. Thiamine, or vitamin B1, is a perfect example of Funk's concept. Thiamine deficiency causes beriberi, a noninfectious neurologic disease that results in loss of sensation, mental confusion, muscle wasting, and paralysis. Now rare, it was once quite common and is cured by thiamine replacement. Scurvy is another good example. Vitamin C, which is ascorbic acid and not actually an "amine," was a frequent cause of death several hundred years ago in sailors during long voyages. It took the British navy close to 50 years to solve the problem. They simply added citrus fruits, such as lemons or limes, to their sailors' diets. This practice dramatically improved the health of British sailors but was mocked by their American adversaries in the War of 1812, who derisively referred to the British as "Limeys."

We have come a long way in our understanding of what vitamins can do for us. In dementia prevention, we particularly need to focus on a few vitamins in the B family. Cobalamin, or vitamin B12, and folate, or vitamin B9, are familiar to many people. Folate, in its manmade form of folic acid, has been a required fortification in cereal products in the United States since 1998. It has successfully reduced the rate of birth defects in the brains, spines, or spinal cords of babies whose mothers were B9 deficient in the first two months of pregnancy. Pyridoxine, or B6, is also important for good brain health.

The B vitamins perform an essential function in your nervous system. They are required for you to synthesize DNA, which is necessary for all your cells and for your metabolism to release energy from the foods you eat or have stored as fat. Deficiencies in these vitamins, especially B12 and folate, cause myelopathy (a nervous system disorder affecting the spinal cord), neuropathy (a disorder of sensation and position, especially in your feet), and depression. And because B vitamins are building blocks for DNA synthesis in all cells, a lack of them can also cause a type of anemia, called macrocytic anemia. This is a condition where your bone marrow makes too few red blood cells and the ones produced are abnormally large and incorrectly formed. The result is too few red blood cells that are needed to carry oxygen efficiently to your brain.

Another complication arising from insufficient levels of B vitamins is a buildup of homocysteine and methylmalonic acid. Putting it simply, when your levels of folate and B12 go down, homocysteine and methylmalonic acid levels increase.

Several decades ago, we discovered that elevated homocysteine levels increase the risk of cardiovascular disease, particularly in men. They do this by increasing the rate of atherosclerosis, in which plaques of fatty material are deposited on the inner walls of arteries. This "hyper-homocysteinemia," as it is called, increases the likelihood of having a stroke and the number of blood clots in your veins and arteries. These strokes and clots, as you have already read, raise your likelihood of dementia later in life. If that were not bad enough, homocysteine, a neurotoxin, interacts with and worsens beta-amyloid, neurofibrillary tangles, and brain shrinkage. Each of these factors is specific to Alzheimer disease. Homocysteine also binds to one of the key excitatory receptors in brain cells called the NMDA receptor. When this receptor is overstimulated, it damages that brain cell as well as those around it.

The Framingham Heart Study 1976–78 cohort showed that when the rate of elevated homocysteine or methylmalonic acid doubled, so did the risk of dementia in this group. On the other hand, if you can lower homocysteine and methylmalonic acid to maintain adequate levels of B12, there is a slowing of cognitive loss. When applied to dementia, elevated homocysteine nearly doubled the rate of dementia in a large-scale meta-analysis combining data from 31 population studies. This relationship was actually higher than the effects due to tobacco abuse. Higher homocysteine levels also predict the onset of dementia in older men and to reduced thinking abilities in women at risk for cardiovascular disease. Because of these and similar findings, elevated homocysteine is now considered a strong risk factor for dementia, which fortunately is also one that can be modified.

Why should your homocysteine level become too high? Part of the answer is that homocysteine is related to stomach acid. You need to have stomach acid for absorption of B vitamins in food. But, as you get older, your levels of stomach acid decline and you cannot access the vitamins in your food as effectively. You may also be taking a medication that reduces stomach acid directly, such as a proton pump inhibitor (PPI). These are sold generically as omeprazole, esomeprazole, or pantoprazole and are readily available without a prescription to treat gastroesophageal reflux disease (GERD). Another common culprit is metformin, an oral medication for insulin resistance and type 2 diabetes. Still other culprits include vegan or vegetarian diets or gastrointestinal absorption problems following gastric bypass surgery. You may even have inherited a vitamin transport defect or developed damage to a metabolic pathway.

What are the best ways to detect these vitamin deficiencies? Your medical provider needs to order specific blood tests for both homocysteine and methylmalonic acid. While most of these providers routinely order B12 and folate blood tests, they do not reliably identify how usable those vitamins become inside your cells where it counts. As a result, about half of vitamin B deficiencies are missed if only a B12 or folate level is checked. The good news is that both homocysteine and methylmalonic acid levels can be lowered with specific vitamin supplementation, guided by your doctor and rechecked over time. Rechecking vitamin levels is important after any supplementation. After all, if your car's oil level was low, you would add a quart and then recheck the level with your dipstick, just to make sure.

Vitamin D is also important. It is a fat-soluble hormone, manufactured in your body, that modulates your immune system to fight disease. It regulates calcium absorption in your gut and helps keep your bones mineralized. It also has a major impact on your brain. Vitamin D deficiency in middle age has been associated with depression and its severity. But it also impacts thinking. Older people with vitamin D deficiency have twice the odds of developing dementia and have many more markers for cerebral vascular disease than people with normal vitamin D levels. Older people who have kept higher vitamin D levels show almost a 25 percent lower risk of dementia. Higher vitamin D levels also activate macrophages, the white blood cells that help your body fight infections and disease, to eat up the beta-amyloid plaques seen in dementia. On the other hand, clinically low vitamin D predicts delirium or confusion while someone is in the hospital for surgery or treatment, as found in one study of over 350,000 elders. This is critically important to dementia prevention, because having an episode of delirium causes greater and faster cognitive decline and earlier onset of dementia.

Some medical providers routinely test vitamin D levels, particularly in geographical locations farther away from the equator, where sunlight is less direct during winter months. Testing for vitamin D insufficiency is also commonly triggered if you report weakness or pain in your muscles and bones. People at the highest risk are older, have darker skin pigmentation, and have inflammatory bowel disease or problems absorbing fats. As with the B vitamins, the best way to assess vitamin D adequacy is with a lab test ordered by your health care provider. Our goal for patients is to have a level between 50–70 ng/mL. One caveat: vitamin D, being fat-soluble, accumulates in the body and can reach toxic levels, which are typically considered 100 ng/mL or above. Therefore, it is important to have your levels monitored by your health professional. Remember the dipstick.

Lastly, we turn to iron deficiency. While it has not been the focus of either large-scale population studies or randomized controlled trials for dementia prevention, iron deficiency is a well-known cause of depression and cognitive impairment. In several thousand patients who were treated in our practice, we found 35 percent showed anemia due to iron deficiency, with a greater prevalence in the older patients. Iron absorption in the small intestine can be impaired by autoimmune diseases such as celiac disease and ulcerative colitis, or following surgery to remove part of the small intestine. Again, the PPI drugs, which lower digestive acid, can also impair your iron absorption. While there is no published evidence on the effectiveness of iron replacement in patients who are deficient (defined as iron- / total iron-binding capacity less than 21% or a ferritin level less than 51%), our clinical experience is that patients improved cognitively when their iron levels were normalized.

As you can see, your dementia risk can be modified by identifying certain vitamin deficits to restore proper levels of these "vital amines." But a word of caution is also in order. Before you go out to the vitamin store and fill your basket with bottles of "all-natural" supplements to kick-start your brain, have a conversation with your health care professional and get your blood tested. Supplementing vitamin and nutrient levels beyond what you need is unnecessary and could be harmful if you over-replace levels that were perfectly adequate.

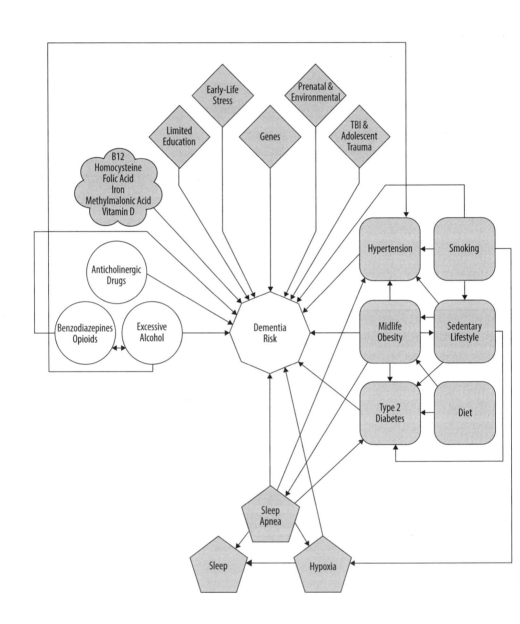

## CHAPTER 8

# Alcohol, Drugs, and Medications

Do you drink alcohol? Chances are that you do. According to US government statistics in 2019, more than half of all American adults drank some amount of alcohol in the previous month and nearly 70 percent in the last year. More than 85 percent have tried alcoholic beverages at some point in their lives. And about one in every four American adults engaged in binge drinking (four drinks for a woman, five drinks for a man within a two-hour period) in the preceding month. Alcohol is extremely popular around the world, with about 2 billion consumers.

Alcohol is also big business and a growth business. Combined sales of all types of alcohol (beer, wine, distilled spirits) in the United States rose consistently from 2011 to 2019, reaching more than 250 billion dollars. Then, in response to the pandemic, consumption in 2020 took another 14 percent jump, likely in response to isolation and emotional distress.

But alcohol use can extend into alcohol abuse, which accounts for nearly 100,000 deaths per year. It ranks third as a preventable cause of death only behind tobacco use and the combination of poor diet and physical inactivity. Roughly 70 percent of those deaths were in men. When you examine the leading causes of death, you discover that medical problems caused by drinking surpass those caused by auto accidents, drug abuse, suicide, child abuse, and falls. That is because alcohol impacts your heart, your gut, your liver, and a range of organs subject to cancers. People who drink have higher rates of hypertension, strokes, heart disease, atrial fibrillation, and cardiomyopathy. They are more likely to get pneumonia. They have gastrointestinal problems including esophageal varices, gastritis, and gastroesophageal hemorrhage. They have liver diseases such as portal hypertension, chronic hepatitis, as well as acute and chronic pancreatitis. They are more susceptible to cancers in the colon and rectum, esophagus, larynx, mouth and throat, liver, and prostate or breast. Alcohol is also a factor in seizure disorders, myopathy or muscle diseases, polyneuropathy or nerve diseases, psychosis, and generalized degeneration of the nervous system.

The number of conditions caused or accelerated by alcohol is by itself surprising. But what should get your attention is that these disorders are the result of only *moderate* alcohol consumption, defined as one to two drinks daily for women and two to four drinks daily for men.

Age plays a role in this analysis because the death rate for these conditions is twice as great for people 65 and older than for those between ages 20 and 34. It is likely that years of frequent alcohol exposure leads to these higher numbers. Alcohol takes its toll on our brains after decades largely because of intermediate medical conditions. Its cellular and chemical damage are often related to diabetes, hypertension, high cholesterol, lack of exercise, obesity, obstructive sleep apnea, heart disease, and stroke.

Not surprisingly, daily consumption of alcohol, even at average levels, is now raising concerns about its being a cause of dementia. But that was not always the case. The early studies in this area were more optimistic. They suggested that moderate consumption was the best choice and possibly even better than teetotalling. These studies showed a J-shaped curve, with no daily consumption carrying a mild risk, low to moderate consumption (one for women, two for men) offering protection from dementia, and any consumption beyond moderate as adding to dementia risk.

In the same vein, a 2020 review of data from the Health and Retirement Study, a nationally representative sample of American adults, examined the alcohol consumption and the cognitive scores of nearly 20,000 people over a period of about nine years. They concluded that low to moderate alcohol consumption was associated with better overall cognition and slower rates of decline. The presumption is that moderate use of alcohol reduces cardiovascular problems and improves BDNF (brain-derived neurotropic factor). However, the study authors caution that the number of subjects who reported high alcohol consumption were few and that chronic medical problems, in addition to excessive alcohol, may be responsible for some of the differences between groups.

Other research has come to a different conclusion. These studies have found that even the "safe" or moderate daily consumption of alcohol causes a faster rate of cognitive loss and could lead to an earlier onset of dementia. Their conclusions are based on studies using brain MRI, where moderate drinkers showed greater brain tissue loss or atrophy as compared to nondrinkers. The MRI scans showed particular deterioration in the hippocampus, a central memory area. The degree of atrophy was dose related: the more alcohol someone drank over the 30 years these people were studied, the greater the loss. People who drank more than the recommended amount of one for women or two for men had nearly six times the rate of shrinkage in the hippocampus and in the corpus callosum, a major communication connection between the left and the right sides of your brain. Such research supports a conclusion that none is better than even one when it comes to daily drinking.

Incidentally, the outcome of alcohol consumption is worse if you have ever experienced a blackout, during which you lost enough alertness that you cannot remember what happened while you were drinking or afterward. Blackout drinkers have a two to three times greater risk for alcohol-induced dementia, according to a 14-year-long study of more than 130,000 middle-aged Europeans. And this may be just the tip of the iceberg. In this well-conducted study, they excluded people diagnosed with Alzheimer disease or vascular dementias and also did not count people who developed any of 14 alcohol-related medical conditions.

Remember those B vitamins from chapter 7? Some drinkers have inadequate levels of vitamin B1, or thiamine, which interferes with the formation of new memories. This is called Wernicke encephalopathy or the Wernicke-Korsakoff syndrome. They also have poor balance and vision. If their thiamine is not replaced and they continue to drink, they will develop dementia and may die. Unfortunately, doctors don't routinely check for thiamine deficiencies, even when they see their patients having balance problems and changes in memory. And many people who drink are aware that their drinking is unhealthy and will hide or minimize their consumption.

Such was the situation with Cordelia. An executive assistant to a financial officer in a major company, this 56-year-old woman unwound after work almost every evening with two vodka and seltzers. She was comfortable with her moderation. We then asked a more specific question: "How do you make your drink?" She explained that she drank half vodka and half seltzer. We pressed on, "How big are the glasses?" And that's when her two cocktails turned into five or six. It turns out that she was pouring into an eight-ounce glass. That's also why, when she inadvertently switched cocktails with her more moderate husband, he swallowed hard and nearly choked. The moral of the story is, if you drink, do the math and be as honest with yourself and your health care provider as possible.

In the end, we believe the evidence that excessive alcohol consumption is a major problem for life, general health, and dementia risk. We, like many of you, struggle to determine if low to moderate use is better or possibly worse than no use. We also puzzle at the contradictory findings emerging from different types of studies, with the neuroimaging evidence supporting abstinence. We will leave it to you to become the final arbiter of which evidence you consider to be most persuasive. We urge you to take a "sober" look at your drinking frequency and volume, as well as when and why you drink. We strongly advise you to avoid excessive and chronic drinking and any binge or blackout drinking. For those who drink to excess or who binge drink, we believe that the evidence is already clear that alcohol is a great problem. As it affects cognition, they can drink or they can think—but not both. For everyone else in this emerging area of research, you should decide what is a comfortable and healthy level for you.

## Benzodiazepines

In 1966, the Rolling Stones exclaimed "What a drag it is getting old." They concluded that every mother needed something to help her calm down, a little yellow pill, a "mother's little helper . . . that gets her through her busy day." They were probably talking about Valium or diazepam, the first in a line of benzodiazepine (BZ) antianxiety and sleep medicines that include chlordiazepoxide (Librium), clorazepate (Tranxene), lorazepam (Ativan), alprazolam (Xanax), clonazepam (Klonopin), and temazepam (Restoril). These medicines are very effective when used for short periods of time and for specific purposes, including as antiseizure medicines and in controlling someone's withdrawal from alcohol. It turns out that alcohol impacts the same BZ receptor site in the brain as do all of the benzodiazepines.

The problem with benzodiazepines is not because you take one before an infrequent airplane ride or to calm yourself enough to tolerate being inside an MRI scan. The problem comes from repeated, chronic use of these BZ medicines. A 2018 meta-analysis combined findings from 19 studies that looked at how benzodiazepines impact specific cognitive functions. It found that long-term users had greater difficulty with their working memory, processing speed, sustained and divided attention, recent memory, and spatial organization. These thinking problems persisted even after the users discontinued taking these medicines. A 2011 study on more than 8,000 people found that the risk of dementia was nearly three times higher for current users of benzodiazepines than for nonusers. Their dementia risk began to decline a month after they stopped the medication, but it did not fully reach the risk of nonusers for more than three years. Another meta-analysis of eight studies in 2016 found nearly twice as great a risk for dementia in their overall sample, although the risk varied among the groups studied.

The starting point for taking benzodiazepines may be very innocuous. A 2021 study of 2.5 million patients discovered that 20 percent who were given a BZ in the context of a major surgery (but had never taken them previously) continued to take these medications beyond the healing period. It is sobering to reflect on how this initiation process mirrors many of the stories about opioid dependence.

While these results are very suggestive of problems for this group of medicines, we want to emphasize a warning to those who are currently taking benzodiazepines: rapid discontinuation can result in severe problems. Please do not go "cold turkey." Any change must be very gradual and done under the supervision of your doctor.

## Anticholinergic and Other Medications

Sometimes the risk for dementia is increased as we try to treat other conditions. Many pharmaceuticals—drugs prescribed by health care professionals—and over-the-counter (OTC) drugs, which do not require a prescription, are anticholinergic. Anticholinergics work against (*anti*) the effects of acetylcholine (*choline*), a neurotransmitter that is necessary for cells within our brains and throughout our bodies to do their work and communicate with each other. As a normal part of aging, your brain's levels of acetylcholine, as well as other neurotransmitters, decline. But they decline to an even greater degree in people who have neurodegenerative dementias, including Alzheimer disease, Parkinson disease, and several others. That is why doctors currently treat memory and cognitive decline in people with dementia by prescribing medications that are "pro-cholinergic." These FDA-approved drugs include donepezil (Aricept), galantamine ER (Razadyne Extended Release), and rivastigmine TD (Exelon Transdermal patch). While each of these medicines works a little differently, their end point is to maintain the existing levels of acetylcholine in the brain. In other words, the drugs we have used for 25 years to treat dementias work in the opposite direction than do many other drugs you take for other problems.

When you take a medication that is anticholinergic, your acetylcholine levels decline and your thinking becomes foggier. You must be wondering why anyone would prescribe these drugs or take them. The reason is that the anticholinergic properties are just a part of the medication's more general action. Their effects on the brain are collateral damage.

In the prescription drug area, three major categories with high anticholinergic properties include tricyclic antidepressants, antihistamines, and overactive bladder medications.

Take overactive bladder (OAB), for example. This condition affects about one in six adults and includes urinary urgency, frequency, and urinary leakage or incontinence. If you complain to your doctor about your bladder, you are likely to be prescribed one of five medicines to reduce involuntary contractions of your bladder. Even though these medications are only significantly effective in less than 20 percent of people, the emotional consequences and lifestyle limitations of OAB will often prompt multiple attempts to control the problem. However, most of these medicines carry an unintended burden for the brain: the same reduction in acetylcholine that helps prevent embarrassing accidents gets in the way of thinking, especially in older age groups where there is already a greater risk for cognitive impairment.

Moreover, the results may not be temporary or transitory. A 2015 investigation of more than 3,400 participants over the age of 65 found that higher cumulative anticholinergic use resulted in higher levels of dementia 10 years later. A 2019 study reached the same result, essentially that the 11-year risk of dementia in middle-aged and older people was significantly greater for those who took more of these anticholinergic drugs for longer periods of time.

You will also encounter high anticholinergic levels in many of the common OTC nonprescription sleep agents that contain antihistamines, such as diphenhydramine (Benadryl). Because sleep problems are extremely common, affecting about a third of Americans, most people are looking for something that works well, does not seem habit forming, and requires no prescription. They often pick up a "-PM" compound that combines a familiar pain medicine that we readily take for a headache or back pain (acetaminophen or a nonsteroidal inflammatory medication) with diphenhydramine. These readily available compounds are often very effective for temporary or transient insomnia. They work so well that you might conclude that you should not risk a bad night's sleep and that it would be better to take one of these pills every night, "just in case." But this is not such a great idea, since you are now setting up a chronic dependency (at least psychologically) on a readily available substance that can truly impact your dementia risk. In addition, anticholinergic effects are additive, with each medicine or preparation contributing potentially to those of others.

But a word of caution before you make any changes to your prescription medicines. You are probably taking a prescription medication for a very good reason, and you and your provider need to be on the same page about your concerns and about your health goals, and especially how to accomplish them safely. Preventing dementia by deprescribing medications is becoming a high priority in medicine today, so you are likely to have a cooperative medical provider when you bring this up for discussion with her.

Drugs are not just additive or cumulative; they can also interact with one another. In the United States, the average person, particularly the average older person, takes between six and nine different prescription drugs on a daily basis. This number does not include nonprescription supplements and OTC medicines. As a result, you can easily encounter a drug–drug interaction, in some cases potentiating or increasing the effect of the medications and in other cases limiting or even negating their effect. When you, as a patient, have several medical specialists who are each focused primarily on their "own" part of your body, make sure that each specialist is aware of what the others are prescribing. Do not assume that each practitioner is reading the others' notes. Remember, they have a large number of patients, but you have just yourself.

To do some more research for yourself, you can also check out the Beers List, short for the Beers Criteria for Potentially Inappropriate Medication Use in Older Adults. Named for its originator, Mark Beers in 1991, it is perhaps the most highly regarded and best-known compilation of medications to avoid in the elderly and in those with specific medical conditions. Published under the auspices of the American Geriatrics Society, it is evidence based and was most recently updated in 2019. It is available as a printable pocket reference card that you can get at https://www.elderconsult.com/wp-content/uploads/Printable BeersPocketCard.pdf. This can also help guide you and your health provider through the extremely complex issues involved in your attempt to mitigate dementia risk.

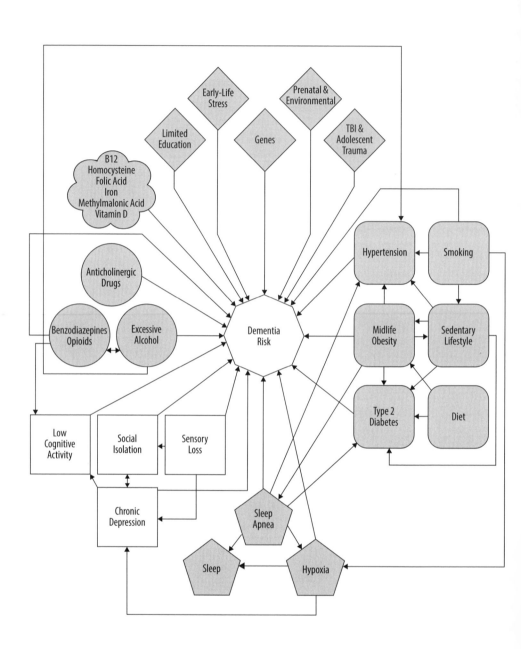

## CHAPTER 9

# Sensory and Emotional Factors That Amplify Dementia Risk

## What Did You Say? Hearing Loss and Dementia

Have you been singing "Hold me closer, Tony Danza" with Elton John all this time? Did you think that Bob Dylan was bragging "The ants are my friends, they're blowing in the wind"? Maybe you thought that Credence Clearwater Revival was suggesting "There's a bathroom on the right." It might have been just a cheap sound system or that your old vinyl was warped by too many revolutions with a bad needle. On the other hand, it may be your hearing.

Hearing loss can impair your ability to think and increase your risk of dementia. As early as 1989, studies were demonstrating that poor hearing was an independent cause for dementia. But, as in many other aspects of dementia, there was little collaboration between neurological specialists and hearing experts, so little research occurred for some years. More recently, large-scale epidemiological studies have demonstrated that impaired audition in midlife accounts for an extra 9 percent of all-cause dementia cases 10 years later. Those who develop hearing impairment are nearly twice as likely to lose cognitive ability. MRI studies show that the brains of people with even subtle hearing loss become measurably smaller in critical areas associated with both hearing and thinking. What makes this even more important is that hearing loss is very common as we age, affecting one-third to two-thirds of individuals who are 70 or older. In fact, the World Health Organization now considers hearing loss as a cause of dementia in up to one-third of cases.

How does this occur? There may be several mechanisms that interact with each other. Both hearing loss and dementia involve the cochlea, a part of your inner ear that translates vibrations of sound into the signals that travel up the auditory nerve pathways in your brain. So, it makes sense that not enough stimulation to the cochlea leads to not enough stimulation to your brain. A second theory posits that your brain is not being sufficiently stimulated by a variety of sounds (think birds singing and music playing), as well as by speech, which conveys both information and emotional tone. Such chronic under-stimulation becomes particularly relevant in noisy, often social environments where sound discrimination is important. This is compounded when your brain tunes out and you withdraw from interactions that on the surface seem unappealing or confusing to you.

A third explanation suggests that the burden of making sense of diminished information overstresses mental capacities and resources. Experimental evidence demonstrates that you really cannot do two things simultaneously as well as you can do them separately, no matter what your teenager tells you when claiming to study algebra with the TV on. Dual tasking becomes an even greater problem as you age, when you don't have as much mental bandwidth. The result is that people with poor hearing have to work harder and use more, often limited, brain resources just to make it through the day. Overall, the interplay between the underlying cellular changes found in dementia interact with decreased hearing to produce the final loss of memory and cognition. As one writer put it, hearing loss is a "second hit" to a nervous system already impacted by dementia pathologies.

While each theory is slightly different, they all lead us to conclude that we may be able to prevent or offset cognitive problems by treating hearing loss through hearing aids or cochlear implants. This is still an emerging area of research, but a 2018 study of 35 older adults with moderate hearing loss was encouraging, finding that after six months those who wore hearing aids had significantly higher memory scores than those without hearing treatment. But the jury is still out on how much long-term prevention benefit can be gained and at what stage of hearing loss will a potential or optimal benefit occur. Some of these questions may be answered by ACHIEVE, a large-scale, multi-center study currently underway. It plans to enroll 850 older adults with mild to moderate hearing loss but without dementia, treat the hearing loss in half of the group, and see to what extent hearing treatment impacts their cognition, incidence of dementia, brain structures on MRI, and quality of life over a three-year period. In the meantime, we advise our patients to get their hearing checked and to consistently wear their hearing aids, even when they are alone. By doing so, they will increase their brain stimulation, enjoy some of the sounds of life, and improve their communication with others. And, if that is not enough of a reason, they will stop believing that "Sweet dreams are made of cheese."

## Seeing Is Believing

Vision loss is also very common in older adults, affecting 18 percent of people older than 70, and it has also been implicated in dementia risk, independent of a variety of other potentially contributing factors. Initially the evidence was cross-sectional, based on comparison rates of dementia between good-vision and poor-vision groups at a single point in time. Then the Women's Health Initiative studied more than 1,000 older women for about four years. Shockingly, vision impairment alone increased the rate of dementia by two to five times. While 8 percent of those with poor vision developed dementia over four years, this occurred in only 3.1 percent of those with better vision. As the magnitude of visual problems increased, so did the dementia rate. Similarly, a 2018 analysis on more than 2,500 adults aged 65 to 84 found that changes in visual acuity predated and heralded subsequent declines in mental abilities. A 2022 study using data from the Health and Retirement Study calculated that "more than 100,000 prevalent dementia cases in the US could potentially have been prevented through healthy vision."

Mirroring hearing loss theories, the underlying mechanisms for decline remain unclear. One hypothesis is that visual impairment and cognition share an age-related pathway. Another suggests that visual deprivation triggers cognitive deterioration, a finding also identified in Parkinson disease patients who develop dementia with hallucinations. Another theory highlights the additional burden on cognitive reserves that results when you cannot see well. Again, these are all potentially compounded by the secondary effects of social withdrawal. One positive note comes from findings of improved cognitive test scores after cataract surgery, suggesting that improving vision could postpone declines in thinking. Prevention of vision loss in middle age is also ranked as one of the most preventable causes of dementia according to the World Health Organization. So, we recommend that you have regular eye health and vision examinations, remediate what you can, and wear your glasses or contact lenses consistently.

## A Double Whammy

What if both your vision and your hearing are going south? Dual sensory impairment (DSI) is estimated to occur in 15 percent of older adults, particularly over age 80. While some research has failed to find any additional burden from DSI in comparison to single sensory loss, a 2020 study of over 2,000 adults found that people with self-reported visual *and* hearing problems were nearly twice as likely to have mental decline when compared to sensory-intact individuals, especially if the impairments were severe. It has also been well established that people suffer from delirium upon hospitalization if they suffer from either sensory impairment, with even higher rates found when patients have DSI. And, as we have pointed out before, delirium leads to further cognitive decline.

## Depression and Social Isolation

As you have been reading this chapter, you probably have also noticed that sensory loss interferes with social connectedness and can cause depression. In 2014, a study of more than 18,000 American adults demonstrated a significant relationship between hearing impairment and mood disorder, particularly among women. These findings were extended by research in 2020 with an equally large population of middle-age and older adults that concluded that vision and hearing problems were separately and together associated with both impaired cognition and depression.

### *Depression*

Depression is often a first sign of cognitive problems, creating some confusion as to whether someone is losing memory ability or is suffering from "pseudo-dementia," a psychiatric condition that looks like dementia. Volumetric MRI neuroimaging studies demonstrate reduction in the size of several key brain structures in both depression and dementia. In addition, one of those key areas, the hippocampus, can be increased in size through treatment with the antidepressant medications sertraline and citalopram. Other research indicates that the depression most commonly seen at the beginning of cognitive decline is less of a melancholia or sadness and more related to apathy or lack of interest. As such, that person's withdrawal from activities that have become too challenging may be the culprit rather than depressive disinterest. It remains unclear if treating depression will slow down or stop a progression into dementia. No matter, in a good workup for reversible and preventable causes of dementia, depression should always be considered.

By itself, depression is implicated in worsening ability to think and greater risk for future cognitive loss. A 2006 meta-analysis of over 100,000 people estimated that depression, especially more severe or recurrent types, doubles your risk of subsequent dementia. In 2010, the Framingham Heart Study published findings that 21.6 percent of people who were depressed at the start of their study experienced dementia 17 years later, compared to only 16.6 percent who had not been depressed. A 2013 meta-analysis combining data from 23 studies also found that mid-to-late-life depression greatly increased the risk of all types of dementia. While these findings were true for Alzheimer disease, the relationship was particularly strong for vascular dementias. This is in line with subsequent research in which the data from more than a half million people showed a clear connection between depression and cardiovascular disease, which underlies vascular dementia.

Researchers have found that neuronal plasticity (adaptive brain function) is impaired in mood disorders and that there are chemical changes in depression that are seen more frequently in dementia, including those involving nicotinic receptors and NMDA sites in the brain as well as increased levels of beta-amyloid protein. But depression is more than a chemical and cognitive condition. It also impacts our relationships.

## Social Isolation

We are social beings. We grow up in families, attend school and work together, pray in groups, watch performances in audiences, participate in sports with teammates, eat meals with family and friends, drink at bars, and gather in interest groups and social clubs. Simply put, we do things together. From childhood and throughout our lives, our involvement with others creates the fabric of our emotional experience and often defines who we are in relation to others. When we are separated from others, most of us struggle. Made abundantly clear by the separation brought on by the COVID-19 pandemic, social isolation is a major factor in depression.

But could the level of social engagement also factor into dementia risk? Longitudinal studies have found a relationship between poor social engagement and increased dementia risk. As a proxy for social engagement, marital status has been studied. A 2019 study found that unmarried adults (widowed, never married, divorced, even cohabitating) had significantly higher likelihood of developing dementia over the next 14 years than did their married counterparts, with a stronger association found in men. But before you run out to a Vegas wedding chapel to protect your brain, understand that such relationships are complex. Take, for example, an equally recent Harvard study of marital status and cognition. They found that married people did relatively well, but so did unmarried (single, divorced) individuals. In their study, it was the widowed group of men and women who more rapidly lost cognitive abilities, particularly if their baseline PET scans had higher Alzheimer disease markers, such as beta-amyloid levels. So, marriage was not protective in that study and, more surprisingly, the widow(er)s were not more depressed than others and actually had higher social engagement scores than married folks.

## Mental Stimulation and Cognitive Reserve

Perhaps the issue of social isolation is unclear because it is not a single entity. Social isolation is complicated by its relationship with the physical and mental components of work, hobbies, and leisure activity. For example, a 2011 study of 235 people over age 75 found that those who participated in group activities outperformed a comparison group on cognitive tests and measures of mental function three years later. But, their social involvement in the writing, exercise, and art activities in this study also involved physical and mental activation in addition to social engagement. While a 2018 English study found that people who watched television for more than 3.5 hours per day had poorer verbal memory six years later, we cannot blame TV alone. We do not know if they would be working or pursuing a more active hobby if they were not watching television so much. It could be that they were more inclined to be socially isolated, avoidant of mental challenge, or physically sedentary.

Working may be cognitively protective. A 2020 cross-sectional study of European women found that those who worked outside the home had higher levels of cognitive function in later life, although coincidentally, part-time workers outperformed those with full-time jobs. An even more recently published study that followed more than 6,000 American women for an average of 12 years discovered that those who "worked for pay" (their definition) in early to middle adulthood demonstrated comparatively better memory functions in later life, regardless of marital or parental status. While suggestive, these study results remain unclear about the specific mechanism(s) that may be operating.

What about retirement? Many people yearn for a time when they can stop working. No punching of the clock, fewer deadlines, greater personal freedom, sleeping in, napping every afternoon, a fantasy of vacation expanded. But, for people who have worked productively and enjoyed working, full retirement may not be so good for their brain.

Large epidemiological studies using populations from Europe and the United States have consistently shown that people who retired at later ages lived longer, had fewer cardiovascular illnesses, and were less likely to develop dementia. A recent Swedish study of more than 63,000 individuals, over a 24-year follow-up period, came to the same conclusion. So don't necessarily give up your job if you want to keep your brain healthy, although you may want to modify your work life.

Consider part-time employment, freelance work, or short-term contracts, what we now call the "gig economy." In the United States, about 10 percent of the workforce falls into this category, with men over age 55 more likely than younger people of either gender. Anecdotally, we know that the ranks of Uber and Lyft drivers, deliverers of everything from auto parts to groceries, security guards, and consultants are often filled by formerly retired workers who "unretired" after a few months. In some cases, they were supplementing their incomes but often they were bored and feeling housebound.

One winter vacation day when we were buying food at a Florida grocery store, a clearly older man was bagging our purchase. When he offered to take the bags out to our car, we balked. After all, he was older than either of us and we were perfectly capable of carrying our own stuff. But he protested that this was part of his job, and it was important to him to get his exercise. That sold us. As we walked to the car, he confided that he used to run a large corporation in the North, but after only a few months of post-retirement golf and noontime poolside cocktails he realized that full retirement was not for him. So, he came to this grocery store where his wife did not shop, minimized his occupational history on his application, got a part-time job bagging groceries, and was never happier. He said that he got to walk miles per day and met the nicest people who were on vacation.

For some people, the question is not "to work or not to work" but rather the quality of the work. Work complexity has been studied in the context of early-life education, later-life social network connectedness, and leisure activities in a theoretical model of "life course cognitive reserve." Cognitive reserve is sort of like your brain's savings account or its "bench strength," to use a sports metaphor. In a Swedish study following more than 2,500 adults over age 60 for a period of 2 to 10 years, higher cognitive reserve translated into lower risk of dementia. For those readers whose work complexity is maximized already or those who have stopped working, you can take heart that the largest contributing factors in this model were late-life social network connectedness and leisure activity levels.

How about building cognitive reserve through brain games—brain training? It rhymes and sounds attractive. Like lifting weights, you could increase your brain's muscle bulk and become mentally more fit. The concept has been so attractive that several companies have created suites of brain games that have been used by tens of millions of people. But not so fast. First, our brains are not muscles in which strength is built by tearing down fibers that then repair and rebuild. While neural plasticity (creating new pathways) is possible, particularly for young people who are creating many more new brain cells than those in middle or later age, it is not likely achieved by practicing specific computerized games.

So tenuous was the data in this area that the Federal Trade Commission, in 2016, fined the creators and marketers of the Lumosity "brain training" program 2 million dollars, alleging that they deceived consumers. According to the FTC's public statement, Lumosity was unable to demonstrate that its games improved users' performance at work or school, or that it delayed cognitive impairment. Although one recent study suggested a modest benefit when such computerized tasks were performed in supervised groups three times a week, the evidence remains weak. Our conclusion is that these games are recreational and may be enjoyable, but research does not show they delay or prevent dementia. As such, we do not include them in our dementia prevention model. Rather than sitting in front of your computer or focusing on your smartphone, you will likely get more benefit from a more social activity. Think Scrabble, poker, bridge, or mah-jongg, games in which you communicate with others and respond to changing game situations.

How about learning a second language or pulling your guitar out of storage? While several studies conclude that bilingual or multilingual people have greater cognitive reserve and delayed cognitive decline, most of these polyglots learned their other languages as children or young adults rather than in midlife or later. Maybe a musical instrument? Several studies find that musicians maintain greater cognitive abilities later in life and that early music training may be protective of speech perception and general cognition in your later years. For second language and musical stimulation, there are theoretical arguments suggesting that they might be helpful. But the scientific literature has so far failed to establish a dementia prevention benefit for either learning a new language or musical instrument in middle to later life.

But this doesn't mean you should not try either a second language or music. It is far better to wear out than to rust out. While the specific evidence for working, engaging in a leisure activity, or participating in music, art, or linguistics is inconclusive, remaining active is psychologically and physically superior to the alternative.

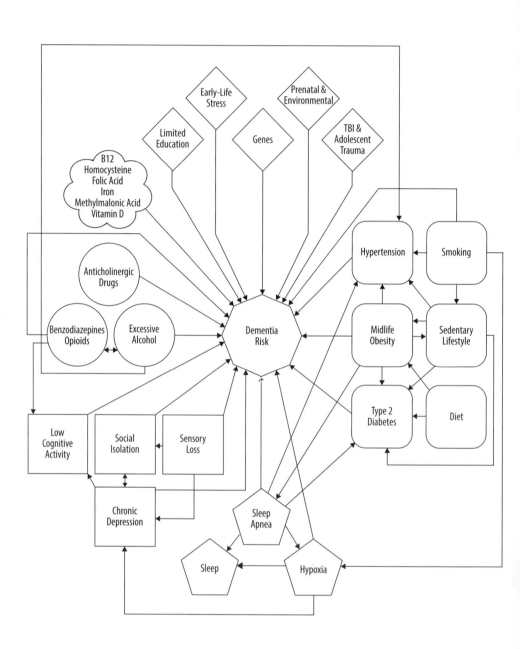

## CHAPTER 10

# Putting It All Together in an Interactive Dementia Risk Model

When all of the elements of our model are shown together, you can appreciate the wide variety of factors that must be considered and the complexity of the associations among these factors.

Looking at this model, you will appreciate that your dementia risk, and therefore your dementia prevention plan, cannot be boiled down to a single factor. No doubt some factors are beyond your control—your genetics, early-life experience, toxic exposure, history of head injury, and educational limitation. But that does not diminish your opportunity to modify their effects by how you care for your current medical conditions, how you manage your weight, whether you smoke, how much you exercise, whether you have vitamin or nutrient deficiencies, if you consume alcohol or depend on sleep aids, and whether you may suffer from common undiagnosed medical conditions such as sleep apnea, sensory loss, or hyperhomocysteinemia.

By appreciating the complexity of these factors, you can also see why no single cure or treatment will work. Numerous studies have examined the role of single factors, such as specific types of diet, exercise, alcohol use, obesity, hypertension, genetics, head injury, and social isolation. In general, they have established suggestive causal relationships between each factor and dementia risk. But none by itself explains enough. Dementia is not a single entity, and no single intervention is sufficient to prevent its occurrence. It will take a more complex approach.

One important multimodal intervention is found in the Finnish Geriatric Intervention Study to Prevent Cognitive Impairment and Disability, otherwise known as the FINGER study. In this randomized controlled trial, they compared two equivalent groups of more than 600 at-risk adults. One group was provided with a multidomain lifestyle intervention composed of diet, exercise, cognitive training, and vascular risk monitoring while the control group received general health advice. Two years later, they found stable or improved cognition for the intervention group in comparison to the control. Their model, shown in figure 10.1, incorporates a number of the factors that we include in our model and, as we will discuss a little later, also shows that timing is important.

The FINGER model is conceptually clear and emphasizes the balance of risk and protective factors in determining the ultimate result, although we believe that it misses some factors that we have included.

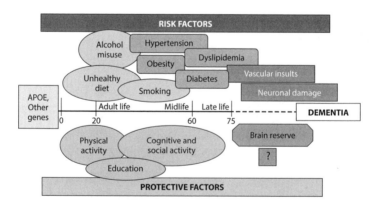

FIGURE 10.1. The FINGER model. SOURCE: Adapted from Kivipelto M, Solomon A, Ahtiluoto S, et al. The Finnish Geriatric Intervention Study to Prevent Cognitive Impairment and Disability (FINGER): study design and progress. *Alzheimers Dement.* 2013;9(6):657–665. Used with permission from John Wiley and Sons.

But in both models, or in any model, the clarity or simplicity obscures a number of background relationships. Dementia risk factors are not simply additive, like the coins in your pocket. They are synergistic, with each element affecting the others.

Here are just a few examples to consider.

## Obesity, Cardiovascular Disease, Diabetes, Sleep Apnea, Inactivity, and Depression

Obesity impacts a wide array of other factors, including cardiovascular disease, diabetes, sleep apnea, inactivity, and depression. As noted in chapter 4, midlife obesity has primary associations with hypertension, dyslipidemia, type 2 diabetes, heart disease, heart failure, and ischemic stroke. But if that were not enough, overweight people have a much higher likelihood of obstructive sleep apnea (OSA) because fat deposits in the neck and elsewhere compress the airway and interfere with diaphragm movement and chest wall expansion, all of which are physical factors that interfere with breathing while you sleep. One study found that even a 10 percent increase in weight increases your risk of sleep apnea by six times! Adding to this, both obesity and sleep apnea interfere with the balance of leptin and ghrelin in your brain. The messaging of these two proteins is disrupted by OSA and obesity. As you saw in the chapter on obesity, this chemical imbalance causes you to have a false sense of being hungry, even though your body does not really need more food right then. We also see a double-whammy effect when insulin resistance is caused by obesity and sleep apnea, resulting in type 2 diabetes, another cause of dementia.

Physical inactivity acts as both cause and effect in obesity and sleep apnea. Overweight people are much less likely to exercise and be physically active. Carrying around a lot of additional weight will tire you out, cause you to move awkwardly and inefficiently, and discourage you from wanting to exercise. Central adiposity (weight in your middle) can also create balance problems and back pain. With less physical activity, overweight people have much greater difficulty burning calories and losing weight, a vicious cycle for sure. Conversely, physical activity helps to reset the point where calories are burned and, according to a 2013 meta-analysis, can also reduce sleep apnea severity even in the absence of weight loss.

We also know that depression plays a part in these relationships. Depression is about 25 percent more likely in someone who is obese, and many depressed people overeat and exercise less. Completing the picture, those with cardiovascular disease also have a higher risk of depression and people with depression are at higher risk for cardiovascular problems.

Some of this loop may also have early-life origins. We know that obesity has an inherited predisposition that is distinct from specific dementia genes. When you add in the importance of prenatal oxygen levels and consider that 15 percent of pregnant women develop sleep apnea during their pregnancy, another element of the model is brought into play.

Lastly, middle-age and particularly later-life depression almost doubles the risk of incident dementia and is associated with poorer general health and much higher rates of cardiovascular and cerebrovascular disease, bringing us back to where we started this section.

## Genetics, Sleep Apnea, Anticholinergic Medications, and Benzodiazepines

Starting from the genetic side of the model, you may have inherited a predisposition for sleep apnea because you have a smaller airway, a less open alignment of your jaw, and a larger body size. Your likelihood of having sleep apnea is about 50 percent higher if you have a first-degree relative (parent or sibling) with this condition. Now add to this predisposition the high frequency of nocturia (arousals during sleep to urinate) in people with sleep apnea and you have disrupted sleep duration and cycles. If you are that person going to the bathroom several times per night because of apnea, you will probably be prescribed anticholinergic medications to increase your bladder control or you will want to take benzodiazepines or over-the-counter anticholinergic ("-PM") sleep medicines. Unfortunately, you now have three combined risk factors for dementia, namely the reduction in oxygen, the depletion of acetylcholine in the brain, and the long-term use of benzodiazepines to maintain sleep.

## Hearing Loss, Social Isolation, Cognitive Inactivity, Chronic Depression, Alcoholism, Sleep Medications, and Smoking

While it is unlikely that hearing loss is caused by these other factors, having untreated hearing impairment will likely lead you to withdraw from social activities because of embarrassment, confusion, and disinterest. Recent research finds that those with hearing loss are even less likely to engage in exercise or even mild physical activity. You may watch TV in a different room because you need a higher volume, avoid answering the telephone, or miss the point of the story or the joke. With poor hearing, you have to work so much harder to decipher the subtleties of a conversation that you don't really want to socialize.

In some cases, a person with subtle hearing loss may become offended by a casual comment. Consider the case of our elderly and age-sensitive aunt, who denied having a hearing problem. She once became very upset during a birthday party while talking with a woman she had not seen in a few years. When that woman asked "How are you?" our aunt *heard* her inquire "How old are you?" And that was a difficult breach in the relationship to repair.

Depression rates are doubled for people with hearing loss, particularly women. In a 2014 study, the percentage of depressed adults with hearing loss increased from 5 percent in those with normal hearing to more than 11 percent in those with hearing impairment. When the hearing loss is subtle, the affected person can be unaware of the change and will instead find the world to be a less interesting place.

Cognitive activity often declines in response to hearing impairment. When you misunderstand directions or responses to your questions, you are likely to experience confusion and arrive at incorrect answers to problems. You may become less productive and avoid contributing to a group discussion, especially while several people are each trying to make a point. Or you may have discovered greater problems when working remotely online.

Alcohol abuse and depression have a high and bidirectional occurrence. People with depression self-medicate with alcohol, a central nervous system depressant. Imagine the effect if you are depressed because of hearing impairment and isolation and then drink excessively to cope with your emotions.

People with depression often have disrupted sleep and begin to rely on over-the-counter sleep medications or benzodiazepines to get through the night, adding a further element of foggy thinking and dementia risk.

Smoking also finds its way into this same cluster of interrelated factors. People with lifetime histories of depression are twice as likely to smoke as those who are not depressed, and some of the treatments for depression show benefit for those trying to stop smoking.

Again, there are genetic and early-life components to many of these conditions as well as contributions from acquired problems such as early-life trauma and head injury.

## Age and Risk Factors

Want even more complexity? At different stages of our lives, certain problems exert greater effects than at others. For example, a single mild head injury in childhood may not result in a difference in that person's dementia risk later in life, while multiple injuries or that same degree of head injury in later adulthood might trigger a significant decline in thinking ability, particularly for someone with already diminished cognitive reserve. Obesity in your 40s or 50s can have a profound effect on thinking but will not affect memory as much if you are already over 70. Sleep apnea in middle adulthood produces cognitive impairment, but if you are already showing cognitive decline in your 80s, your dementia may be causing your sleep apnea, not the other way around.

At a 2010 State-of-the-Science Conference on Preventing Alzheimer's Disease and Cognitive Decline, sponsored by the National Institutes of Health, Dr. David Bennett emphasized the "complex relationship between genetic and environmental factors that lead to disease progression and neurodegeneration" and presented a table of these factors separated by the time period in which they occurred: intra-uterine, early life, midlife, and late life. As a simple example, high body mass index in midlife increased the dementia risk while low body mass index in late life had the same effect. As often true for life in general, timing is important.

When these and other additional interrelationships are considered, the model we present at the top of this chapter becomes almost too complex to consider. It begins to resemble a tangled knot.

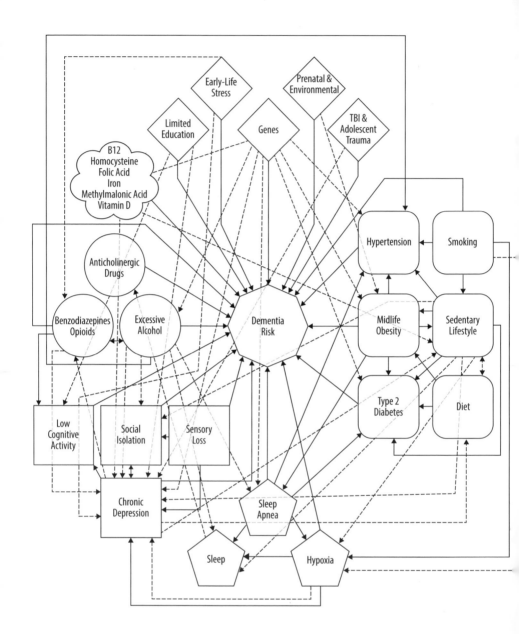

# Is Dementia Risk a Gordian Knot?

According to legend, Alexander the Great and his conquering armies entered the Phrygian capital of Gordian (in modern-day Turkey), in 333 BC. There, they encountered an ancient wagon that had belonged to

King Gordius, the father of King Midas. The wagon's yoke was covered by a large and tangled web of knotted ropes. According to a prophecy, whoever could unravel this knot was destined to rule all of Asia. Alexander, determined to conquer Asia and the rest of the world, repeatedly attempted to untangle this knot, but without success. Undeterred, he declared that it was not important how the knot could be undone but only that it was undone. He drew his sword and sliced the knot in half! Having undone the Gordian knot, he then marched on with his emboldened legions to conquer the defending armies.

Like the Gordian knot of ancient times, the knot of dementia risk has many varied and interrelated medical and behavioral strands. But, unlike Alexander, we have no great medical or magical sword. No dietary regimen, brain game, vaccine, infusion, or pill is able to cure or to prevent dementia. No single intervention will cut through your individual knot. With no all-powerful sword available or even on the horizon, your dementia risk knot must be untangled.

As you will see in the next chapter, your knot is unique. To get you started on your personal approach to untangling it, we have developed an inventory that will help you to identify your ropes and their knots. After you have completed this inventory, you will be in position to identify some of your problem strands and decide which knots you can begin to untangle first.

Do not be discouraged. While untangling can be a frustrating endeavor, your knot is really just an accumulation of separate threads. Many can be loosened and some can be undone. We will give you some unraveling ideas and what you learn by untying parts of your knot will help you in other parts of it. As we promised in the Introduction, if nothing else, each of these elements will help you to improve your health.

# PART III

## Where You Stand and What You Can Do about It

## CHAPTER 11

# Your Dementia Prevention Checklist

So far, we have discussed dementia prevention factors in the abstract. And, as you have seen, there are a great number of them and many of them are interrelated. While interesting theoretically, you are hopefully much more interested in how these variables impact your health specifically, in other words, "What are my risk factors and what can I do about them?"

To move us from abstract theory to action, we have constructed a survey for you to take, presented in the form of a checklist. The completed checklist is your own personalized profile of strengths and weaknesses. We have limited the checklist to those factors that are modifiable and for which there is solid evidence. In other words, genetic loading, history of childhood trauma, and adolescent football or soccer concussions are not part of this survey. Those are in the past while our focus is your future.

## How to Complete the Checklist

We have divided the checklist into six sections, each containing between two to nine questions. In all, there are only 23 items. You should circle your best response for each item. This will place your answer into one of four possible categories: On Target, Near Target, Off Target, and Don't Know. Some of the responses require a numerical answer, such as a laboratory value. Your "numbers" will determine into what category you fall. Other responses are descriptive, requiring you to best characterize your behavior or lifestyle when answering. You will notice that some categories have more leeway and will allow you to see that you are in the Near Target range. Other questions have no middle ground: you are either On Target or Off Target. Please try to use only one option for each question. If you do not have enough information right now, select the Don't Know option.

**MORE DETAIL ABOUT THE OPTIONS**

· On Target means that you are in line with the goal or best practices in that area.

· Near Target means that you are close but not quite there. For example, your blood pressure may be slightly high, your weight 10 pounds more than desirable, your vitamin D within "normal" guidelines but not optimized for best results.

· Off Target indicates that you are currently farther away from the target than you want to be, putting your health at risk now, as well as later. A good example would be a blood pressure of 160/120 or if you are smoking cigarettes.

In choosing *Target* as the defining term, we have purposely avoided value terms, such as good or bad. Our goal is to guide you in obtaining important facts and objective information about your own modifiable dementia risk factors, not to alarm or shame you. On the other hand, we are not willing to water down the science to the degree that it becomes meaningless. If, for example, you are presently overweight, the bottom line is that your metabolism is storing too much energy in the form of fat and is less fit than it was intended to be; those extra pounds you are carrying are raising your risk for a number of medical conditions directly tied to dementia.

Here is another point of information as well as a disclaimer: This checklist and all of its information is presented as a guide; it is not intended as medical advice. It does not replace personalized advice from your own health care professional, someone who knows you and can factor in all of your possibly complex health information. Additionally, your age, gender, race, and other health conditions will impact some target ranges. Treat this like a GPS: even though it says to turn right, you might be driving in a tunnel, not on the street above.

Now it is time to take the next step in decreasing your dementia risk by completing your individual Dementia Prevention Checklist.

There are three ways for you to do this:

1. You can turn the page and begin.
2. You can open the camera app on your phone or digital device and hold it up to the brain-shaped QR code shown below. The QR code will take you to an online interactive checklist that you can complete on your phone or device and print out for later reference.
3. You can also find the checklist at www.braindoc.com.

Either way, completing this checklist can be the first step in using your head to save your brain.

# Your Dementia Prevention Checklist

## *Labs*

| FACTORS | DON'T KNOW | OFF TARGET |
|---|---|---|
| Homocysteine (Hcy)<br>Must be interpreted with MMA | ☐ | > 10 µmol/L |
| Methylmalonic acid (MMA)<br>Must be interpreted with Hcy | ☐ | ≥ 0.23 µmol/L |
| Vitamin D-25 OH | ☐ | 0–30 ng/mL |
| Total Cholesterol<br>HDL<br>LDL<br>Triglycerides<br><br>Target levels depend on age, health, risk category | ☐ | Not applicable |

## *Drugs/Medications*

| FACTORS | DON'T KNOW | OFF TARGET |
|---|---|---|
| Anticholinergics and nonprescription sleep medications | ☐ | Frequent use currently and high ACB score—assess risk/benefit ratio |
| Benzodiazepines | ☐ | Daily or most days of the week for more than 90 days |

## *Cardiovascular and Breathing Conditions*

| FACTORS | DON'T KNOW | OFF TARGET |
|---|---|---|
| Type 2 diabetes (T2DM) and insulin resistance | ☐ | HbA1c ≥ 6.5<br>and depending on other medical conditions |

| NEAR TARGET | ON TARGET |
| --- | --- |
| Not applicable | < 10 µmol/L |
| Not applicable | ≤ 0.23 µmol/L |
| 31–49 ng/mL | 50–70 ng/mL |
| Not applicable | < 150 mg/dL<br>≥ 60 mg/dL<br>≤ 71 mg/dL<br>≤ 150 mg/dL |

| NEAR TARGET | ON TARGET |
| --- | --- |
| Episodic use currently—assess risk/benefit ratio | Not used or infrequently used currently, low ACB score |
| Small doses a few times per week for less than 90 days | None to infrequent |

| NEAR TARGET | ON TARGET |
| --- | --- |
| HbA1c = 5.7–6.5 and depending on other medical conditions | HbA1c = 4.5–5.6 and depending on other medical conditions |

## Cardiovascular and Breathing Conditions (cont.)

| FACTORS | DON'T KNOW | OFF TARGET |
|---|---|---|
| Hypertension (high blood pressure) | ☐ | > 130 / > 90 and depending on other medical conditions |
| Sleep apnea | ☐ | AHI ≥ 5.0<br>5–15 = mild<br>16–30 = moderate<br>31+ = severe |

## Habit and Lifestyle Practices

| FACTORS | DON'T KNOW | OFF TARGET |
|---|---|---|
| Alcohol consumption | ☐ | Female: 2 or more per day<br>Male: 3 or more per day<br>Any binge drinking |
| Tobacco, particularly cigarettes | ☐ | Any |
| Obesity | ☐ | BMI > 30 |
| Exercise | ☐ | Sedentary activities, little to no walking, casual housework or golfing with a cart |
| Sleep | ☐ | Sleeps less than 5 hours or more than 9 hours per night, insomnia or interrupted sleep, frequent nocturia, sleep "behaviors" |
| Diet | ☐ | High in processed or fast foods, sugars and carbohydrates; low in vegetables and legumes |

| NEAR TARGET | ON TARGET |
| --- | --- |
| Not applicable | 120/80 |
| Not applicable | AHI = as close to 0 as possible with treatment or 0–4.9 without treatment |

| NEAR TARGET | ON TARGET |
| --- | --- |
| Not applicable | Female: 0–1 per day <br> Male: 0–2 per day |
| Any | None |
| BMI = 25–29.9 or < 18.5 | BMI = 18.5–24.9 |
| 20–30 minutes moderate exercise most days, some weight or resistance training | 30–60 minutes moderate exercise every day, some weight or resistance training |
| Sleeps 5–6 hours per night, occasional insomnia, nocturia 0–1 times per night, awakens refreshed most days | Sleeps 7–8 hours per night, very occasional insomnia or interruption, nocturia 0–1 times per night, usually awakens refreshed |
| Episodic good diet | Diverse diet with olive oil, vegetables, legumes, low in sugar and simple carbohydrates |

## Habit and Lifestyle Practices (cont.)

| FACTORS | DON'T KNOW | OFF TARGET |
|---|---|---|
| Viral or infection avoidance | ❑ | Few or no vaccinations, disregarding public health policy advisories |
| Dental hygiene | ❑ | Irregular or no visits to dentist, little or no brushing and flossing, periodontal disease |
| Injury prevention | ❑ | Little to no use of seat belts in car; helmets on motorcycle, bike, skis, skateboard; cane or walker if falls risk. Acts impulsively. |

## Social, Emotional, and Cognitive Factors

| FACTORS | DON'T KNOW | OFF TARGET |
|---|---|---|
| Mental stimulation | ❑ | Very little. Not engaged—time spent napping, TV, repetitive tasks, "puttering" in house. No work, few hobbies. |
| Social engagement | ❑ | Seeing few friends or only family, living alone; withdrawn and isolative |
| Stress management and coping | ❑ | Frequently anxious, worried, depressed, feeling out of control; conflicted relationships |

| NEAR TARGET | ON TARGET |
| --- | --- |
| Some age-appropriate vaccinations, episodic attention to public health policy advisories | All or almost all age-appropriate vaccinations, consistent attention to public health policy advisories |
| Regular dental visits, but irregular brushing and flossing for periodontal disease | Regular dental visits, daily brushing and flossing to minimize or avoid periodontal disease |
| Inconsistent use of seat belts in car; helmets on motorcycle, bike, skis, skateboard; cane or walker if falls risk | Consistent use of seat belts in car; helmets on motorcycle, bike, skis, skateboard; cane or walker if falls risk |

| NEAR TARGET | ON TARGET |
| --- | --- |
| Reading, playing games alone, assembling puzzles, knitting, sewing, working in shop or on car | Actively engaged in school, job, volunteering; learning new skill, language; engaged in art, playing music, interactive games, attending classes |
| Attend religious services, sometimes going to senior center, see friends or family occasionally, own a pet | Actively participates in organizations, clubs, social or religious groups; regular contact with friends and family; engaged and interactive |
| Occasionally anxious, worried, depressed; would like to feel more in control; adequate relationships | Feeling content, fulfilled, safe, able to meet challenges; strong relationships |

## Sensory Impairments

| FACTORS | DON'T KNOW | OFF TARGET |
| --- | --- | --- |
| Hearing | ☐ | Tests as impaired and refuses hearing aids or declines testing despite urging; needs high TV volume; expects others to speak louder and repeat themselves |
| Vision<br><br>Ophthalmic examination frequency depends on age and medical conditions | ☐ | Poor vision but refuses to wear glasses or contact lenses |

# What to Do Next with the Findings

Start by examining your Don't Know column. This is often the most important category because many dementia risks are due to unidentified problems. For example, your homocysteine and methylmalonic acid levels could be too high, reflecting inadequate availability of critical nutrients for brain cells and blood vessels to work the way they should. The same is true for vitamin D or other abnormalities. You cannot drive a car if the gas cannot get into your engine, regardless of how much is in the tank or how good you are at driving. So, getting these levels checked is important.

| NEAR TARGET | ON TARGET |
|---|---|
| Hears well in most situations; problems in crowded social situations, on phone, or noisy places; wears hearing aids selectively, usually not when alone | Tests as normal or appears to have intact hearing or has impaired hearing and wears hearing aids consistently (and has hearing and assistive devices checked yearly) |
| Mild visual loss, avoids glasses or wears glasses inconsistently | No visual loss or corrects for visual loss by wearing glasses consistently |

Perhaps you have undiagnosed sleep apnea. Because poor oxygenation of your brain reduces your brain's ability to make energy and interrupts the normal pattern of sleep stages needed for restorative sleep (to some degree because it causes you to get up and urinate three times every night), you are constantly tired, maybe even cranky during the day, you hate to exercise, and you just want to lie on the couch. So, knowing if you have this controllable problem has widespread benefit.

And if your hearing is impaired, you may not even be aware of how much you are missing, but your brain is under-stimulated in several critical regions and reduces its ability to change and learn, not to mention that you no longer find pleasure in socializing or in playing cards.

So, your first task is to see if you can fill in some blanks.

# Labs (Blood Tests)

*Homocysteine.* This amino acid is an active co-factor in the production of the energy molecule ATP. It should be measured in conjunction with methylmalonic acid levels. Homocysteine can be affected by moderate-to-severe kidney disease, hypothyroidism, smoking, certain psychiatric and cancer drugs, and alcohol use. When elevated, this amino acid reflects an inherited or acquired problem with our cells using vitamin B9 (folate) and/or B12 to create ATP. Elevated homocysteine is an independent and potentially reversible cause of dementia, and it increases the risk of cardiovascular disease as well as decreasing how easily blood vessels can dilate when there is a greater need for blood and oxygen. When high, homocysteine indicates decreased production of ATP. This condition is an independent risk factor for dementia.

*Methylmalonic acid.* This substance is an intermediate step in the production of ATP and the most sensitive test to determine the adequacy of vitamin B12. A deficiency in B12 is an independent cause of a potentially reversible dementia.

*Vitamin D-25 OH.* This test is the best indicator of vitamin D availability in our body. This vitamin is actually a hormone and has a powerful role in our immune status and affects cognition, mood, energy, pain, and bone strength. While "normal" laboratory values can be as low as 25 ng/mL, target values for brain health are much higher.

*Cholesterol.* A type of lipid, or fat, which is an essential part of all cells, cholesterol is the raw material from which our body produces steroid hormones, like estrogen and testosterone, as well as the stress hormone cortisol. There are several types of cholesterol: high-density lipoprotein (HDL; "good cholesterol"), which is protective and low-density lipoprotein (LDL; "bad cholesterol"), which can cause cardiovascular and cerebrovascular disease.

If any of these blood tests have not already been performed and recorded in your medical record, you will need a "lab slip" or have an electronic order from your primary care provider to go to a laboratory where they draw blood samples for medical testing. These are commonly associated with doctors' offices or are in hospitals. Depending on your age, your health history, and your relationship with your health care provider (HCP), this may be as easy as a phone call or as complex as an office visit coupled with persistent persuasion by you (the health care consumer) showing that you really need to know the status of these indicators.

Some providers will view this as a very positive sign because it signals your investment in good health. Unfortunately, some HCPs may view these blood tests as an unnecessary expense to the health care system and may try to persuade you that you don't really need it. But what you don't know *can* hurt you, and you deserve to understand what is going on in your body. If you meet with resistance to these tests, we suggest that you emphasize your interest in protecting your brain and your desire to have a positive partnership with your provider. Such a positive and committed message signals your commitment to your health rather than dissatisfaction with their care. Also, please feel free to share our chapter on the important role played by vitamins and nutrients in brain health.

## Drugs and Medications

*Anticholinergic burden (ACB).* Anticholinergic medications block acetylcholine, an important neurotransmitter in your central and peripheral nervous systems, and interfere with your brain working effectively. Acetylcholine levels decline as we age. People with Alzheimer disease, dementia associated with Parkinson disease, vascular dementia, as well as other conditions are known to have even lower amounts of acetyl-choline in their brains. Consequently, preserving existing acetylcholine is a target for several dementia medications. However, many nonprescription sleep aids, allergy medications, and cold preparations are very "anticholinergic." They typically contain a class of drug called an "antihistamine," such as diphenhydramine (Benadryl). But while they are helping you sleep or drying up your runny nose, they are also depleting your brain of acetylcholine. In addition to the antihistamines, many prescription drugs have anticholinergic properties, including older "tricyclic" antidepressants and medications for urinary incontinence, Parkinson disease, COPD, and some GI conditions. The effects of these medications are cumulative, so that each one separately may not have such a great impact on acetylcholine levels but the totality of them do. One goal of intervention is to reduce or "deprescribe" medications high in anticholinergic levels or find alternatives that do the same job but are less centrally anticholinergic and create a less negative impact on your brain.

So how do you measure your anticholinergic burden (ACB)? At least eight different online calculators are available for you to determine a medication's ACB and its theoretical impact on your brain. Find an online calculator (for example, www.acbcalc.com). Find the generic or brand name from each of your prescription and regularly used nonprescription medications and enter them into the calculator. If the drug has an anticholinergic effect, the name will drop down from the list. Click on it and you will see its severity-of-effect score, from one to three. If the name does not drop down, its ACB is zero. You add up the scores to determine your Total ACB. If it is out of the target range, discuss alternatives to the prescription medications with your health care provider and consider whether you can reduce or eliminate your use of over-the-counter preparations.

*Benzodiazepines.* Benzodiazepines (BZ) are prescription drugs indicated for the treatment of anxiety, uncontrolled seizures of any cause, and alcohol withdrawal. Some prescription sleep medications also belong to this class. Common BZs include Valium (diazepam), Librium (chlordiazepoxide), Xanax (alprazolam), Klonopin (clonazepam), Ativan (lorazepam), and Restoril (temazepam). This class of medications is habit forming and has high abuse potential, so that the longer someone uses it the more they need to take in order to get the same desired effect. Long-term use of BZs (more than 90 days) is known to cause cognitive impairment. If you are using this class of medication and want to discontinue it, you should only do so under the supervision of a health care provider. Do not stop a BZ "cold-turkey" as this can be dangerous.

## Cardiovascular and Breathing Conditions

*Hypertension (high blood pressure).* Blood pressure is the pressure of circulating blood on the walls of blood vessels when your heart beats (systolic) and the pressure when your heart rests between beats (diastolic). It is measured using a blood pressure monitor on your upper arm or wrist. Your health provider has very likely recorded your blood pressure at one or more visits. You may be able to check this, as well as your lab reports, by going to your online records or by calling your provider's office. Be aware that different blood pressure devices can register different blood pressures on the same person, and that blood pressure varies by the physical position you are in, your activity level just before your pressure reading was taken, the time of day, and your anxiety level ("white coat syndrome"). If you are planning on taking your blood pressure regularly, consider using the same automated cuff at the same pharmacy or grocery store each time, or consider buying one.

*Type 2 diabetes and insulin resistance.* T2DM is a chronic medical condition that affects the way sugar (glucose) is metabolized by your body. When this condition is present, cells no longer have an effective response to insulin, the hormone that is needed to bring glucose inside cells to produce energy, or ATP. People with T2DM may actually be making more insulin than someone without the condition, but their cells are resistant to the effects of the hormone, which is why the earliest stages of this condition are referred to as "insulin resistance." There is a genetic basis in over 70 percent of people who have this condition, which decreases life span and increases risk of dementia. We measure the body's response to insulin by checking the glycated hemoglobin in the blood, the HbA1c level. This represents an average of how "sugary" the red blood cells are over the past 90 days. Depending on your age and other health conditions, your doctor may have checked this in the last year. If not, now is a really good time, regardless of your age, gender, or weight. Find out your number.

*Sleep apnea.* Inadequate air flow to lungs while sleeping results in oxygen deprivation to your brain, called obstructive sleep apnea (OSA). This is tested by a polysomnogram (PSG) or overnight sleep study, which monitors your breathing, heart rate, oxygen levels, and sometimes your brain waves. The study produces a score called the Apnea Hypopnea Index (AHI), the average number of times your brain is deprived of oxygen each hour while you sleep. Let's look at a mild case of OSA, which is represented by an AHI between 5 and 15 per hour. This score is the equivalent of someone holding a pillow over your face to stop air from getting into your mouth and nose, kind of like being smothered, 5 to 15 times every hour. When air does not get to your brain, brain cells die. You are unaware of this, in most cases, and will likely protest that "I sleep just fine." But remember, you are asleep. Other people, especially bed partners, are often much more aware of your snoring, gasping for breath, multiple small awakenings, and excessive movement as your body tries to adjust to take in more air. So don't dismiss their concerns. On the other hand, you may sleep alone or your partner may sleep so soundly that they are unaware of your symptoms. But the diagnosis is based on objective results from an overnight sleep test, not a survey of symptoms or bed partner report.

Fortunately, there is very effective treatment for this condition. The gold standard treatment is Positive Airway Pressure (PAP), which when used consistently through a variety of PAP devices (CPAP, BiPAP, ASV) will often produce improvement in your energy and cognition and will delay progression to dementia for people who already have mild cognitive impairment.

You can start this conversation with your provider by downloading the STOP-BANG Sleep Apnea Questionnaire. By simply answering eight yes or no questions, you can get a rough idea of your risk of having OSA. In addition to STOP-BANG results, please tell your doctor how many times you get up in the middle of the night to urinate (nocturia) or if you have headaches, especially upon awakening, because the STOP-BANG does not include these classic and cardinal symptoms of sleep apnea. Use this information as a springboard to ask your health care provider to order a sleep study. You may be able to do this test in your own home if you don't have a serious heart condition. As you have seen in chapter 5, sleep apnea is a critical aspect of dementia prevention and is well worth the test.

## Habit and Lifestyle Practices

*Alcohol.* Take an honest look at your drinking habits. Remember that one drink is calculated as 12 ounces of 4.5 percent alcohol beer, 5 ounces of 12 percent alcohol wine, or 1.25 ounces (one shot) of 70 proof hard liquor. Many craft brews have a higher alcohol content, and many lite beers are lighter in calories but not so different in alcohol content, so the math remains unchanged. One more thing: like many people, you may pour liquor with a heavy hand and without using a shot glass, so make the adjustment in your calculations.

*Tobacco use.* Smoking or vaping of tobacco products (4 mg eLiquid = 1 pack of cigarettes) is the standard measure. The question here is very simple: Do you smoke?

*Obesity.* Please step on the scale. It is just a number. You can then calculate your body mass index (BMI) with a free online calculator by filling in your weight and height.

*Exercise.* Count any type of moderate cardiovascular exercise that raises your heart rate. Include brisk walking, running, swimming, biking, tennis, yoga, and tai chi, as well as resistance or weight training. Sometimes stretching counts. Yardwork that is physically active can also qualify, but don't count sitting on your riding mower or playing golf if you ride in a cart.

Housework and gardening are always a question. For some people these can be a true workout, with a lot of physical activity, but for others their more sedentary and languorous approach doesn't provide much benefit. When looking at exercise, pay attention to and record what you actually do—not what you did in the past, what you wish you did, or what you plan to do. You can download a pedometer calculator app for your cell phone to record your steps and distance. You can also use a wearable device such as Fitbit.

*Diet.* Everyone has different advice about diet. Results are inconclusive with respect to any particular food, or combination, or calorie count specifically preventing or delaying the onset of dementia. For a complete discussion, please refer to our chapter, and just keep in mind sugars, simple carbohydrates, and trans fats are really not good for anyone's brain.

## Social, Emotional, and Cognitive Factors

*Mental stimulation.* Keep it interactive, favoring tasks that require problem-solving, thinking in new ways, and skill development. Emphasize new activities and new learning and new events and new opportunities. "New" stretches the brain and creates new synapses, those lovely connecting points between neurons that are the basis of your brain's ability to grow and stay young. Doing things in new ways (eating with the other hand, driving to work differently) is a start, but you need much more than that to create new pathways. Avoid periods of inactivity or falling back into the comfort of repetitive overlearned activities that keep you in a mental rut. Learn a new language, play a new musical instrument, try a new approach to a problem, start a hobby, take an online or in-person course, or volunteer for a community-based event or activity. You may even want to take a part-time job, especially if you can develop or use a new skill.

*Social engagement.* Involvement in organizations, friendship groups, clubs, family activities, preferably with face-to-face involvement constitutes social engagement. Ideally, physical contact is desirable, although virtual engagement may be a necessary alternative. Being married or in a long-term relationship helps, but don't do this just for dementia prevention.

*Stress management and coping.* A subjective sense of well-being, feeling safe, being in control and able to make your own choices, maintaining an optimistic outlook, adapting to change and challenges, and dealing with loss are all critical to taking good care of your brain. You may benefit from meditation, yoga, and other forms of self-care. Even if you've never considered it before, you may want to think about professional support, as in counseling or psychotherapy. Having an objective, outside person with whom you can share your concerns can make them more manageable. Often just the process of putting feelings into words makes them easier to understand and manage. You may also benefit from psychotropic medication if you realize that what worked for you before isn't quite cutting it now.

*Safety.* Your balance while walking and exercising is important. If you've been falling or tripping, don't keep this a secret. Discuss this with your health provider who can order relevant medical tests and possibly a physical therapy evaluation to determine the cause and potential treatment. Most of all, you do not want to fall and injure yourself. Having a head injury or bone fracture can land you in a hospital and possibly eventually in a nursing care facility. Consistently use seat belts and avoid speeding. Some accidents are not preventable, but the extent of injury from these accidents may be modifiable. And, please, do not drink and drive a car.

We urge you to follow public health warnings, particularly in this age of pandemic diseases, to get vaccinated against transmissible illness, and to be cautious regarding tick bites and mosquito-borne illness. While these types of advice make good medical sense, they are also very important in dementia prevention because injuries, infections, communicable diseases, and the emergent hospitalizations and complications that result from them accelerate cognitive decline. Good safety practices make good sense.

## Sensory Impairments

*Hearing problems.* Don't assume that everyone else is mumbling; get tested by a well-trained audiologist. Some hospitals and university medical centers have audiology departments. The VA offers this service in some locations. Even some of the big-box wholesalers, like Costco and Sam's Club, provide these exams as well. If you have an objective hearing loss that can be improved by hearing aids, we urge you not to ignore this problem. The most recent research suggests that hearing loss may be one of the most easily modifiable factors in dementia prevention.

*Vision problems.* See an ophthalmologist, a medical doctor specializing in the eye, who can measure your visual acuity and also examine you for underlying visual changes that cause blindness and for which treatment is indicated. Such conditions include glaucoma, macular degeneration, and cataracts. Problems with our eye health are often related to underlying vascular factors and lack of oxygen. Decreased visual acuity, despite correction, is an independent risk factor for dementia.

# For People Currently Experiencing Cognitive Symptoms

Up until now, most of what we have discussed focuses on prevention. What if you are already experiencing cognitive problems? In addition to the medical factors previously highlighted, if you are already experiencing cognitive changes, your doctor should order additional tests. These include iron-to-total-iron-binding ratio and ferritin, thyroid tests, triglyceride levels, C-reactive protein (CRP), erythrocyte sedimentation rate (ESR or sed rate), brain natriuretic peptide (BNP), a complete blood count with differential (CBC/diff), tests for venereal diseases (RPR or VDRL and FTA-ABS), HIV, IGF-1, Chem 7, and liver function panel. You do not want to leave stones unturned, especially if treatment can improve your thinking ability or delay decline.

While having all of these tests for inflammatory disease, anemia, infections, cancer, autoimmune diseases, heart failure, high cholesterol, endocrine disorders, hearing loss, and sleep apnea may seem like overkill—and will result in extra work on your part and numerous vials of blood—each of these could reveal a reversible or modifiable cause for your thinking problems. Remember, this is all about prevention and ultimately will result in a lot less work and a lot less expense than searching for a treatment or a cure.

## What Next?

Look at your On Target areas. We hope there are many of these. You can congratulate yourself and take a mental victory lap. While some of these may be due to good genetics, excellent parents, or simple luck, others represent good health choices you have made. You may have chosen never to start smoking or to limit how much alcohol you drink. But other On-Target ratings are the result of changes you have already made. These can help to inform you about how to make changes in the areas where you are not so strong. Maybe you have succeeded because of support from a coach or trainer. Maybe you are competitive and lost 40 pounds because your best friend lost 39. Maybe you heard a talk, read a book, or had a conversation with someone you trust and decided that their advice made a lot of sense.

Reviewing how you successfully quit smoking, started a regular exercise program, changed your diet, or decided to purchase hearing aids may give you valuable information that will help you achieve changes in the Off Target and Near Target areas you have identified.

Change is hard. You already know how difficult it can be to alter your existing and well-worn habits, patterns, and beliefs. But just because it is hard does not mean that it is not worth doing. In the next chapter we will explore why making change is hard to do.

## CHAPTER 12

# Everybody Wants to Feel Better, But Nobody Wants to Change

Old Joke: "How many psychologists does it take to change a lightbulb?" Answer: "Just one. But the light bulb really has to want to change."

Change is a major issue for most of us. Helping (motivating, coercing, facilitating) change in ourselves and others is one of the primary factors in medicine and personal health care, but also in consumer buying behavior and in public health care (think vaccinations).

As you just completed your Dementia Prevention Checklist, you hopefully found a number of areas where your health and behavior are already On Target or at least Near Target, requiring some relatively small tweaks and adjustments. Congratulations. We know that you may have had to work hard to hit some of the targets.

But you probably also discovered one or more Off Target, more worrisome items that can increase your later-life risk for dementia. You also know that at least some of these are not accidentally Off Target. They are the result of your longstanding habits, behaviors, and choices. You now see that, if you truly want to prevent dementia and protect your brain, you might need to make some changes! You may have to stop doing something you really enjoy or start doing something you might not like. You might need to use a CPAP machine, modify what and how much you eat, start and maintain an exercise program, use a weekly pill box to avoid missing doses, reduce how much alcohol you drink, get a hearing test, or go to bed earlier.

And now you are faced with a dilemma: you can either decide that those Off Target areas are not so important or you can decide that you need to make some changes. You are faced with a hard fact: making changes to old patterns is very difficult and may even seem unfair. Like everyone, you want something that is quick and easy, a simple tweak, a small adjustment, a shortcut, what they now call a "life hack." If only you could reduce your dementia risk by making a few changes to your diet, adding some vitamins or spices, or taking a pill that you can buy without a doctor's prescription to "support brain health." Who would not want something that is easy and immediate—just add water and stir? But here's the dilemma: if it was that quick and easy you probably would have done it already based on your own sound judgment and likely the advice of your doctor. If you had done it already, you probably would not be reading this book.

While there is some truth to the quip that "everyone wants to feel better, but nobody wants to change," it is certainly overstated. Some people seem to make positive changes easily. We have all heard stories of a life-enhancing midcourse correction that someone made without any problem. Someone who had an epiphany one day and threw out their cigarettes, poured every ounce of alcohol down the drain, became an avid practitioner of yoga, or took up long-distance running—some inspiring person who ditched years of unhealthy habits in one fell swoop! In retrospect, when you hear of their accomplishment, they made it look so easy that you are tempted to jump on their bandwagon. Maybe they have a "method" or a line of food or vitamins that gave them the ability to overcome their inertia and reach their goal while barely breaking a physical or emotional sweat.

In reality, those people are rare and definitely not like the rest of us. We, as well as you, struggle to change our habits and patterns of behavior that have developed over a lifetime.

# Why Is Change So Hard?

We will highlight three factors that make it hard for us to effect important and lasting change:

1. Repetition and familiarity
2. Fear of the unknown
3. Cause-and-effect discontinuity

## *Repetition and Familiarity*

Repetition, much like muscle memory in athletics, is very good for maintaining new habits but is part of the reason that you have become very attached to your current habits. You have simply done them time and again. They are familiar and may have become a defining part of who you are. "This is the way that I do it" could be emblazoned on your T-shirt. You may have difficulty explaining why you do it that way, only that you have always done it that way. Up until now, you think it has worked. And, because of a psychological principle called cognitive dissonance, you will discount any evidence suggesting that it has not worked (you are out of breath walking upstairs, you fall asleep during movies, you spend 300 dollars a month on cigarettes and need three inhalers). Cognitive dissonance makes it hard for you to accept any information or opinions that run counter to your habit. Instead, you will seek out data or anecdotes that support your position. You will laughingly recall the times you made it home from a night out but cannot remember where you had been. You recall your uncle who lived to be 100 while smoking a pack of Lucky Strikes every day. You have heard that some people who are very overweight have normal blood pressure and blood sugars. And then there was your friend's grandmother who lived to a ripe old age without ever doing anything more physical than housework.

Cognitive dissonance was a big part of the thought process for our recent patient, a 70-year-old woman with obvious hearing problems. After she asked us to repeat our questions five or six times in just the first 10 minutes of our interview, we mentioned that she might have hearing loss. She surprised us by responding that the audiologist she saw, more than a year ago, had reached the same conclusion! *Why no hearing aids?* we wondered. "I just can't see myself wearing hearing aids" was her only answer. Her answer was firmly entrenched despite our informing her that hearing loss was now considered an independent cause for dementia, that hearing aids might improve her current memory and thinking, and that she might better enjoy being around other people if she accurately understood what they were saying. Marshalling our best persuasive arguments, we kept approaching her resistance like an oyster shucker looking for a weak spot in a bivalve hinge. No, she was not concerned that someone would see the hearing aids. No, it was not the cost. It wasn't even that she had a bad experience with hearing aids in the past. Her best answer: "This is just the way I am, and I don't want to change."

Hopefully this is not you, because your history of repetition and your cognitive dissonance may overwhelm your willingness to make changes that your brain deserves. It is hard for any of us to change and will take your awareness, commitment, problem-solving, and some creativity.

## *Fear of the Unknown*

Like many of us, you may fear things that are new to you. You forget that much of your life has involved dealing with new and unknown experiences. Like it or not, you have been changing since you were a child. Many of these new experiences reflected your growth, independence, and success. From your awkward attempts to roll over, then stand, and eventually run and jump, you changed your behavior. Graduating from training wheels, swimming without floats, getting to stay up later, going off to school, sleeping over at a friend's house, and starting a job or military service. All of these were changes. You probably took these changes for granted and did not consider that it was only as a result of your change in habits and routines that you were able to grow and become more competent. The changes you made seemed so natural, so normal, and so expected that you overcame your fear of the new and unknown. You also did not fully recognize that each step was somewhat of an experiment. To make it to the next level successfully, you had to try out new approaches, learn from your failures, and continually modify your behavior until you eventually hit the target. While it started in childhood, it continued throughout your adolescence and into adulthood and parenthood.

Some of what made these changes okay was the fact that many people before you had done the same things, although maybe not in exactly the same circumstances (who knew, in 1980, that we would be this involved in social media and digital devices today?). But there was enough of a roadmap that you could follow it as you grew. Thank goodness, because change is the essence of growth and development. It is also the key to survival. Organisms that cannot change and adapt to new environments don't thrive and will eventually die, only to be replaced by those that can adapt and change. This basic element of

Darwinism cannot be overstated. Survival of the fittest. Change is the essence of survival.

But somewhere in time, particularly in middle age to later life, you may have forgotten this lesson and instead developed resistance to change. You became "set in your ways." Your habits and patterns became crystallized. "I am fully cooked" exclaimed one of our patients as she resisted changes to her habits at age 45 that were likely to protect her brain at age 65 or 75. Although she had gotten to this point in her life successfully and had hit all of the physical, social, academic and occupational milestones, she had stalled out in midlife. Making changes now seemed threatening, something to be avoided. She, like many of us, wanted to rely on existing habits and rituals, those over-learned and well-practiced behaviors that felt comfortable. For her, they had become "the way I do things." The foods she ate, the activities she pursued, her social interests, the type of clothing she wore, even the route she took to the store became engrained as rituals and habits. In her mind, these habits were the essence of who she was. So, as she saw it, making a change in habits risked losing herself, her identity. No wonder that she put on the brakes and dug in her heels.

She was probably afraid of newness, but she may have also been afraid of feeling foolish. After spending 30, 40, or 50 years doing something one way or believing something, you might feel foolish to change your behavior or your mind. It could feel as if you had lived your life stupidly up to that point. Who would want to admit to that? It would be like the character in the old TV commercials for V8 juice who realizes all too late "I could've had a V8!"

Nobody wants to feel foolish, and we certainly do not want to suggest that your health habits are an index of a life poorly lived. But you may be living on automatic pilot or cruise control, doing the things you have done forever, with little thought to their effects. Every once in a while, you can experience an opportunity to rethink those habits, decide if they still work well for you, and put yourself in a better position to move forward. As you will see in the next chapter, sometimes discovering new information or a technique you can use to become more successful will prompt you to make a change that works out better than before.

In the meantime, it can be helpful to explore how you developed your habits.

## How Do Habits Develop?

Some habits began as an imitation of your parents, what psychologists call *modeling* or *imprinting*. In a classic experiment, ducklings hatched in the presence of a dog followed the dog as if it were the parent. You are not very different. You look to those who raised you. They were a lot bigger than you, took care of you, and seemed to know what they were doing. They were also the ones telling you if you were doing it correctly. As a result, you learned "the right way" to hold a fork, knife, and spoon (ever notice how people do this somewhat differently?), what words to use when you needed to empty your bladder or bowels, how to care for your body, how to deal with conflict, and how to manage frustration and stress. You learned a lot about food preferences, activity levels, and habits from your folks. You were young and accepted most of this unconditionally. Over time, you viewed those habits and preferences as being "normal." If your Off Target habits began that young, there may be a lot of readjusting you will have to consider.

Peer modeling is also partly responsible. You were looking for a road map to being successful as a child and adolescent. What better way to do this than to watch what the older or apparently more successful kids were doing? Maybe the "cool kids" were smoking, so you struggled not to cough or pass out from your first cigarettes until you could smoke with the best of them. You wore your clothes and combed your hair a certain way, used language that only kids like you understood, and embraced a set of habits in order to fit in and feel connected. This may have led you to develop good study habits and an attitude of caring for those around you or it may have directed you to hang out in the woods and binge drink or do daredevil stunts with your all-terrain vehicle.

Some behaviors are developed through demonstration and instruction (this is how you hold a baseball bat), some through emulation (this is what the TV stars are wearing this year), and some you created, on your own, by superstition (bounce the ball three times before every foul shot). Pay attention to your rituals and you may discover that you unconsciously always put on your left sock first when getting dressed, that you always shave one side of your face first, or that you always salt your food before you taste it. "Where did I learn to do this?" you might ask. Even though you cannot give a good answer, you are likely to persist in doing the very same things over and over and to find it uncomfortable to do them differently. Emulation and then repetition make for pretty powerful habits.

We are not saying that you should throw out all of your habits and patterns. Some habits and rituals work very well. You can think about other things while you drive to work if you always go the same way, even though it might take longer. Women of childbearing age can remember to take their birth control pill every day by keeping the container next to their toothbrush. And the fact that there are 28 pills in the container (even though 7 of them are made of sugar) tells us that repetition helps to maintain consistent behavior. By automatically putting on your seat belt when you first get into your car, just as a habit, you will dramatically increase your chances of surviving an accident. Ritually putting your keys or phone in the same place may save you hours of searching over the course of your life.

Some habits, on the other hand, cause problems. Maybe you typically eat a bowl of ice cream while watching TV, take a nap when you get home from work rather than taking a walk, pick up fast food at the drive-through because it is a weekday and you don't want to cook after classes, or have a couple of cocktails before dinner, just as a habit. Or maybe you take a Xanax every morning "just in case" you encounter an anxiety-provoking situation. These automatic and repeated activities can inadvertently lead to obesity, sedentary behavior, and overdependence on substances, each of which elevates your dementia risk.

Another related problem is that many habits can be adequate in the short run but may not work as well in the longer term. You probably could stuff yourself as a teenager without gaining a pound, while the same tactic in your 50s fails because of the midlife decline in your metabolic rate. Running can be a great exercise in earlier life but much harder on your body as you age. Customs, rituals, and survival techniques that worked adequately for 50 years can work against you for the last 30 years of today's typical lifespan. As you look ahead to those next 30 or more years, you could benefit from an improved game plan.

## Cause-and-Effect Discontinuity

In general, much of human behavior is governed by cause and effect. People are programmed to do what feels good and avoid what feels bad or causes pain. While that seems simple enough and rather obvious, a major factor in this equation is that of "timing." They say that timing is everything in life. In this case, the time lapse between cause and effect is a major reason that makes it difficult to motivate you to change a habit today that will not affect you for some years to come. The more closely in time the effect follows the cause, the stronger the connection. The more distant the consequence, the weaker the connection. Immediacy, or a very short interval between cause and effect, is a key ingredient in developing any lifestyle habit, but it particularly works against you when the habit feels good now but is bad for you later.

Part of this is due to your brain's neurochemical release of dopamine and other neurotransmitters when you experience momentary pleasure, whether it is an exhilarating ride at an amusement park, an illicit drug response, the taste of a delicious food, or the attention of someone who you find particularly attractive. These releases of pleasure chemicals in your brain, whether endogenous (created internally) or exogenous (created externally), keep you coming back even when other parts of your brain warn you off.

As a simple example, let's take food. When you taste something and find it appealing, you want to eat more of it. Many foods that are high in salt, sugar, and carbohydrates taste great and very immediately spike your dopamine release and your blood sugar levels, causing you to feel happy and comforted. So, you like to eat them. They may also be part of what you learned in childhood as a way to reduce your stress or anxiety ("You look upset. Here, have a piece of cake.")

But while the pleasure part of the habit is quite immediate, the negative health effects are delayed. Imagine how different it would be if you gained weight within an hour of eating too much or if you ate something that had too many calories or carbohydrates! On the other hand, imagine if you lost weight the hour after you chose a different food or skipped that extra snack. You would probably always stay at your healthy weight goal because the feedback would be so immediate that you would regulate yourself. If you are salt sensitive and your blood pressure immediately rose while you were enjoying the potato chips or pretzels, you would probably cut back. In the same way, if you could see immediate positive outcomes from exercise, alcohol moderation, or skipping a cigarette, you would have little difficulty embracing healthier habits.

But, as you well know, it does not work that way. The delay between what you are doing and what it is doing to you is separated by time to such a degree that you do not easily make the connection between the habit and your health, only between the habit and your immediate pleasure. Consequently, you keep doing what feels good now.

We deal with pain in the same way. You will not keep your hand for very long on a hot stove unless your peripheral receptive nerves aren't working. You pull away due to pain before you experience tissue damage. In this case, the immediacy is very beneficial. But suppose that the cause–effect interval was extended because you had type 2 diabetes and peripheral neuropathy and you had lost a lot of the sensation in your feet. You could walk around with a nail in your foot, or you might stand on a hot coal that dropped from a charcoal grill without any awareness until you ended up with an injured foot or an infection.

In the world of dementia prevention, most of the cause-and-effect relationships are distant or disconnected. Overeating, smoking cigarettes, binge watching TV while lying on the couch, or drinking a six-pack of beer are activities that generally feel good now but cause problems later. On the flip side, getting a flu shot, having a dental cleaning, or hitting the gym don't usually give us a lot of dopamine release right now but yield significant health benefits later. It makes a lot of sense that many of our dementia risk-raising behaviors include easier, less demanding, more immediately rewarding activities. Habits that are healthier are often harder and less pleasurable right away.

## Medical Advice for Change

Your doctor has very likely informed you, perhaps chided you about some of your health habits, such as the dangers of overeating, lack of exercise, excessive drinking, any drug use, and cigarette smoking. And, in today's climate of broadly disseminated health news and warnings written or pictured on product labels, this is not exactly news to you.

You really do know the risks. But, unless you are having symptoms or your health has raised really large red flags (suggesting likelihood of illness or death), you may not have heeded this information. It is like the research experiment some years ago that found markedly increased commitment to treating sleep apnea only after people watched a video of themselves struggling to breathe while they slept. Otherwise, and even when watching other people with sleep apnea struggle, you might not see the risk as being very real and certainly not immediate.

At your physical, you have probably been polite—"I know, I really should . . . (lose weight, cut down on alcohol, get exercise, or wear a seat belt)"—in response to your doctor's advice. You may smile sheepishly, acknowledge the value of the advice and the helpful spirit in which it is given, but leave it in the doctor's office along with your paper exam gown when you leave. Such advice remains an external and abstract goal. In other words, you have not owned the concept because someone else has told you that you "should" do it. In your mental framework, it remains "my doctor wants me to," rather than "I want to." These types of external goals only have persuasive power within about 30 feet of the doctor's office or 30 minutes from the time of the appointment. They quickly fade away until the next visit (which you may postpone if you have not changed your behavior).

It is also quite possible that you have sincerely promised your doctor you will "try" to change. But "trying," just like the proverbial New Year's resolution, is often half-hearted, short-lived, and likely to fail. We hear a lot about "trying" in our office. When one of our patients promises to try to change some behavior, we do a demonstration of "trying" with them. It is an easy demonstration that you can do right now. We place a piece of paper on the table and ask the person to try to pick it up. When they pick it up, we tell them "No, this is not correct. You picked it up. We want you to *try* to pick it up." Eventually they realize the point of the demonstration, that "trying" occurs when someone makes an attempt and fails. Ultimately, we recommend that you follow the sage advice given by Yoda from *Star Wars*: "Do or do not. There is no try."

## Owning the Change

As you have seen, there are a lot of reasons why change is hard. Yet, change continues to be essential no matter how old you are, how firmly you are set in your ways, and how much you don't like to change. But perhaps you can now begin to reconsider change, with your new understanding of how some of your habits and attitudes developed and how you may have become resistant or set in your ways. We will also present some psychologically sound, research-based change techniques in the next chapter. Alas, there is no magic here, but there are approaches based on cognitive science and psychology that we have found helpful in over 40 years of therapeutically coaching behavior change in our patients.

The process for you begins by answering the question that you will hear in motivational talks: "How badly do you want it?" When it comes to your brain's future, you hopefully will answer, "A lot!"

New Joke: "How many psychologists does it take to change a reader's behavior?" Answer: "None. But the reader can if they really want to change."

## CHAPTER 13

# Use Your Head to Save Your Brain

One of the most amazing things about your being human is your ability to imagine what could be, to consider multiple and future options, choose a desired outcome, and then put a plan in place to achieve that goal. You can use the powers of your neocortex, the "new brain" that controls language, imagination, planning, and higher order thinking, to counteract some of the effects of cause-and-effect discontinuity, as discussed in the last chapter. You can use images, concepts, and beliefs that you can hold in your mind to change your behavior. This process of setting goals and labeling them is part of what we call cognitive psychology.

Cognitive psychology is the study of mental processes—how we think. Cognitive behavioral therapy (CBT) is derived from cognitive psychology and is a method used to help people better understand and change their behavior. The major principle of CBT is that your feelings and the behaviors that result from your feelings do not occur randomly or exist in a vacuum. Nor are they caused directly by outside events. Instead, CBT teaches us that your feelings and your actions depend on how you think and interpret events or the actions of others.

This concept is often surprising. Like many people, you may think that you just "have" feelings or that your feelings are caused by how other people act. "She made me angry" or "I just felt that way" are common statements. But they are actually untrue. Nobody causes you to feel any way in particular. Other people just act. They do things. How you feel depends on how you interpret those actions. When you see, hear, or otherwise perceive the actions of others, you interpret their actions through your own beliefs and life experience. In other words, you "view" the world not as it is but rather by mentally looking through your particular "lens" of interpretation. Another way of saying this is that your thoughts form a "frame" around a mental picture, just as an artist places a frame around a painting to enhance it. How the picture is framed and where it is hung will influence how you view it. A child's drawing hanging on the refrigerator is "cute," but what if it were framed and hung in a museum of modern art?

In psychology, where there are no experts to define the value of painting, the frame does a lot more than surround the image, it often determines how we interpret it. Imagine this situation: You are riding on a packed subway car at rush hour. Everyone is standing so tightly crowded together that you cannot easily look down. Suddenly you feel a rather firm poke in your side. You wince, slightly. How do you feel? When we ask people this hypothetical question, about half say that they feel angry and the other half report fear. Almost nobody is indifferent. Then we examine what they are saying to themselves, how they are interpreting the event. Those who are irritated will explain that they are thinking, "How rude! How dare someone invade my space!" The fearful imagine that someone is about to rob them and has placed a knife or gun in their side.

We then ask each person to imagine that they look down and discover that the other person is a blind nun, who inadvertently jabbed them with her cane. Using that new interpretation, "seeing" the same situation through that new perceptual lens or mental frame, the angry may feel guilty and the frightened feel relieved. Almost nobody feels the same way even though they were certain that their feelings were based on the experience itself. As you think about this, please notice that nothing about the situation itself has changed. The subway is just as crowded, the jab just as firm and unexpected. What has changed is your interpretation of the event and, therefore, your emotional response.

This basic illustration of your thoughts interpreting an event and leading to your emotional response is fairly clear-cut. But many situations in life are more complicated than this and the feelings you experience are more nuanced and complex. Suppose you have worked with the same coworkers on an assembly line for years. One day you are offered a promotion. Is joy your only response? Maybe. For while the promotion is rewarding and the money is better, you may also feel sadness at the prospect of losing your buddies (now that you are the boss), fear that you might not make the grade, and maybe even some anger that you had to wait so long for such a well-deserved promotion. In any case, it is not a single feeling. But regardless of its complexity, how you feel is based on what you think.

A cognitive behavioral approach does more than explain how our feelings develop. It also offers you some important tools that you can use to engage your brain to change your behavior. Here is a 10-step process that you can use as a model to make an important change.

## 1. Identify an area for change

Let's look at your Dementia Prevention Checklist from chapter 11 and pick something to work on. Maybe you should choose a Near Target behavior. The chance of success is high because not a lot needs to be changed. If you already walk 20 minutes most days, adding another 10- to 15-minute walk is not a big change, but it can make a difference in your fitness and possibly your strength and your weight control. If you have already cut down to a half pack of cigarettes from a previous two-pack a day habit, you can now plan a strategy to further reduce and eliminate cigarettes from your life. Even a small health behavior, like flossing your teeth or taking a daily medication to control your blood pressure, diabetes, or depression, can make an impact when you increase your regularity of doing it. Small does not mean insignificant. Making small changes incentivizes you to make others and these add up to some important gains.

You may want to start bigger because you discovered that you have a number of Off Target areas that may be connected, as you saw in chapter 10. This happens often in the area of vascular risk factors. The number of Off Target areas may cause you to feel disheartened about whether you can make progress. Do not despair: the interaction of these areas means that making a positive change in one can bring about a positive change in others. The rule is to start somewhere but not everywhere. Nobody can work on everything at once. Quell that temptation to tackle a total renovation of your physiological "house." Start in one place, in "one room," achieve some degree of comfort and mastery there, and then use that success to expand from there, in a progressive way, just as if you were actually cleaning your house.

## 2. Set specific goals

Vague and general goals go unmet. Being healthier or more physically fit is nice to say, but you need to state the general terms *healthy* and *fit* in more specific terms in order to translate your desires into action. Traditional medical professionals often drop this ball because they frame their advice too generally, in terms such as "You need to lose some weight and exercise more," or "You should not be drinking so much." This leaves their patients confused about where and how to start. True behavioral change requires more tightly defined goals that are connected to a purpose. You need to spell out exactly what you want to achieve and the actions you need to take in order to reach it. And, as any good salesman knows, the sale should be connected with a benefit.

Consider such goals as these:

· I will reduce my carbohydrates to less than 15 grams per day, because if I do this I will lose some of my excessive weight, be able to get back into my size 8 clothes in six months, or reduce the chances that I will experience dementia like Mom.

· I will do 10 pushups every morning before I step into the shower, because if I do I will build muscle in my chest and arms, eventually get rid of my love handles, and fit back into my jeans so that I will like the way that I look.

· I will buy my cup of coffee each morning at a different place where they don't sell such wonderful pastries so it will be easier for me to lose another pound or two this month.

· I will get off the couch when I feel sleepy and get into bed with my CPAP mask on so that I will get more hours of breathing while I am sleeping and this will help to keep my brain cells at their best.

· I will do a quick relaxation exercise when I begin to feel stressed instead of reaching for a Xanax or beer to help reduce my anxiety, so that I will develop control over my anxiety and preserve my brain.

## 3. Expect and foresee obstacles

Everyone has obstacles that have prevented them from hitting their dementia prevention goals. If you did not have obstacles, you would already be On Target, at your brain health goal—like the highway sign near the new housing development says, "If you lived here, you would already be home." Truth is that we all have obstacles, and many of these we have created ourselves. Some of these may be hidden or subconscious. But many are there for you to see if you pay closer attention. Most of us know our tricks, our hidden secrets, our cheats and workarounds. You may not be proud of them, but they exist. Identifying them gives you the chance to better manage them. Consider the following examples.

You know that you will not get to the gym if your feet first touch your home doorway at the end of a busy day. Like it or not, it is true. Use that knowledge and make sure to drive home via a route that goes past the gym, even if it is out of your way. Then, you are much more likely to stop, even for a brief workout. And, most of the time, you will extend that brief workout (after all, you are already there and starting to sweat) until you do the workout that you feel proud about.

You know that you snack at night because it feels good then. You do this routinely even though you feel guilty the next morning. Good diets begin at the grocery store. So don't go to the store hungry and don't put those snacks into your cart. You tell yourself you are just keeping those chocolates around "in case of company," but you also know that you become the "company" after your spouse goes to bed and only you are watching.

Do you like to smoke after you have had a few beers? Don't go to places where you can smoke if you really want to tackle this seriously. Again, start at the store and don't buy cigarettes so you are even less likely to go someplace where you can smoke.

Since you often forget your dental appointment, record your appointment in your phone as soon as you make it. Don't promise yourself you will record it when you are less busy. And set a reminder for a few days in advance so that you can change any competing appointments.

By foreseeing obstacles and recognizing how you often defeat your best plans, you can change your approach and ultimately your health.

## 4. *Examine your* but

No, not *that* butt. We are talking about the *but* that is part of your obstacle. It is the *but* that you think to yourself or say aloud about half-way through your response when someone suggests that you do something new. There may also be a *should* before it, such as "I know that I *should, but* . . ." The part of the sentence that follows your *but* is likely what has prevented you from reaching your goal.

You agree that you should take a walk *but* you are too busy, tired, or unmotivated. Your doctor wants you to stick to a diabetic diet *but* it seems like a lot of work, you have a sweet tooth, or it takes time at the end of a busy day to cook so you will "have" to get a fast-food meal. You hate the fact that you smoke, *but* you have been doing it for years, have failed several times to quit, and you have a really stressful meeting tomorrow.

As you examine your *but*, you may recognize that you have no evidence for these statements and that many of your reasons are untrue or unnecessary. Are you really too busy to take a 10-minute walk? What exactly is a sweet tooth except an acceptable shorthand for you to rationalize that you enjoy eating sugary foods? And why does your history of failed attempts to quit smoking stop you from quitting now? You know that socializing is important for cognitive and emotional health. Are you really too introverted to join a club or group? And taking on new mental challenges improves your thinking. Are you really too old to learn a new language? Do you really need to keep smoking because your partner does? When you examine your *buts*, you will discover that these are critical obstacles that you have erected and that you can tear down. As one of our patients laughingly noted about her diet, "If I examine my *but* now, I may have less butt to examine later."

## 5. Take baby steps

While many people first heard this term in the 1991 comedy *What about Bob?* in which a patient tracks down his psychotherapist during the therapist's vacation, the concept of taking small steps to achieve a longer-term goal is very important. And very old. Ancient Chinese philosophers are credited with advising, "A journey of a thousand miles begins with a single step." The advice holds true today. Any change in what we do or how we live must start by taking small steps and making minor changes consistently in order to be successful.

The first rule is to start. As soon as possible. Procrastinating, waiting for a perfect time, and delaying the first step means you will often fail to start. And make sure that you start small. We can trace many failed attempts to change to excessive ambition, not apathy. No matter how hungry you are, you cannot (and should not) eat your entire meal in one bite. In the same way, while you hate to see the number on your bathroom scale, you cannot change your weight in one day or one moment. In fact, when you think about it, why do you put your scale in the bathroom? What can you do there to change your weight? Shouldn't it be in the kitchen where it might help you to make a different choice?

Moderation is the key to success when you want to make an achievable change that will last. Nobody safely loses 30 pounds in one month by dieting. Nobody reshapes their physique in one week even by exercising for hours on end. If you try to go from couch potato to distance runner in one week, you will probably end up back on the couch, but this time with an ice pack or a walking boot. Maybe the only exception to this rule is addictive behavior, in which small steps are not within your control.

Success in taking small steps depends on choosing a better initial goal. Losing 10 pounds in six months makes great sense. Cutting down on your portion size, eliminating that bedtime snack, and buying different foods are an even better goal. Choosing smaller goals, and connecting them to the behaviors that lead to those goals, will make a difference and are repeatable over time. You can start today by making some changes in when, how much, and what you eat. Ten pounds in six months is less than two pounds per month, less than a half pound per week, just a couple ounces each day. Just a couple changes in your behavior. This is a repeatable and sustainable process, not a flash in the pan that will reverse itself when you can't stand to be deprived any longer.

As we will discuss later, exercise is much the same. Walking 10 minutes three times per day will begin to meet your cardiovascular goals without injury or major lifestyle modifications. Doing just a little more, progressively, over time will get you to lifestyle goals and, even more importantly, keep you there for the long run. To update the ancient philosophers, "Life is a marathon, not a sprint."

## 6. Use the just-noticeable difference, or JND

In the 1850s in Germany and England, before Alzheimer and his colleagues were slicing up brains and examining them microscopically, a group of early psychologists, known as psychophysicists, were studying perception and sensation. They were looking at how people experienced the physical forces in their environment. They wondered what it would take for someone to perceive if an object was heavier or lighter or if a sound was louder or softer. In this group, physiologist Ernst Weber developed the concept of the just-noticeable difference (JND), what has come to be called Weber's law. The JND represents the least amount that something must change in order for a person to notice there being a difference at least half the time. Weber discovered that such sensory discrimination is based on mathematical ratios: the difference must be greater if the baseline property is larger.

For example, suppose you have a 10-pound weight. When you add that to the 25 pounds that you lift when doing a bicep curl, you will clearly notice the difference. It will feel much heavier and you will probably struggle. However, if you had added that same 10 pounds to the 150-pound bar that you can lift easily with both hands in a chest press, the weight will probably not feel heavier. It is below your JND. So, 35 feels far heavier than 25 but 160 does not feel greater than 150. Turning up the heat by 5 degrees in a 175-degree sauna probably falls below your JND, but you will feel much warmer by turning up the heat by 5 degrees in a chilly 60-degree bedroom. Optometrists use this same principle when determining the strength of your eyeglass lens. "Is lens A better or worse than lens B?" becomes the perceptual question.

Psychology has made little use of the JND, except in the applied field of marketing and advertising. A candy manufacturer wants to boost profits while not increasing price or losing customers. The company wonders "how much smaller can I make this candy bar and still charge the same price?" The same principle applies to the number of ounces in a cereal box or the minimal amount of material when making a discount piece of clothing. Conversely, when the manufacturer wants to show off an improvement in a product, those "newer, brighter, larger, faster" elements of their product, they need to figure out how much change they must make to make the difference apparent.

So, what does this have to do with your behavior change? Piggybacking on the baby steps idea, suppose that you want to improve your level of exercise but want it to be as painless as possible. If you are exercising 10 minutes every other day, going to 20 minutes each day will feel like too much. But how about filling in the days when you don't exercise? What if you take a 10-minute walk every day? You probably will not notice a difference, but this will double your weekly exercise. Or how about eating snacks from a smaller bowl? The bowl still looks full and you will probably not mind the difference. You will feel as fulfilled but you will have eaten less. In behavior therapy we help people to approach frightening situations, such as phobias, by starting just below their JND of fear. If you are afraid of dogs, you cannot pet a dog, but you probably can look comfortably at a cartoon of a dog. After becoming comfortable with that, looking at pictures of puppies sleeping may now fall below your JND of fear. Soon you can watch puppies playing, then adult dogs walking, and gradually you become comfortable petting the same friendly dog that sent you into a panic just a few weeks before. When taking baby steps that are just below your JND, try to be creative and experimental in finding where the point of changed perception occurs. In this way, you can use your head to ultimately improve your brain.

## *7. Play it where it lays*

This golf axiom is adaptable to cognitive behavioral psychology as well. Avoid wishing you were at a different starting place. Some people give up before they begin because they believe it is too late. They rationalize that they have been smoking, drinking excessively, overeating, avoiding exercise, or failing to care for themselves for so long that making a change now will have no effect. Their *but* is, "I am so old and set in my ways. How can this help now?" Our honest response is that we do not know how much it will help, but we are very sure that doing nothing will never help. And very often, the *but* overstates the permanence of the damage. The very fact that you are reading this book suggests that you retain some hope for a better future. So, no matter where your ball has landed on (or off) the course, we encourage you to start where you are, to play it where it lays.

## 8. The rest stop: Take a break and check out your surroundings

Because most health habit changes require persistence over time, making a periodic check-in can help you to see how far you have come and where you need to go. In our work with people who have cognitive decline, periodic retesting of their memory and thinking abilities helps to determine how effective our approach has been and what new steps to take. If you plan for these "rest stops," you can adapt your plan more effectively.

If you have ever tried to lose weight by dieting, you know that you often lose weight initially and then reach a plateau. Your metabolism has adjusted to your new food intake level and you can't seem to lose another pound. Your frustration rises and you become fatigued. What first seemed new and shiny about your diet change, what first seemed to be the answer to your weight loss woes, now feels like a dead end.

It is time to take a one-day holiday! The important word in that phrase is *one*. Recognize that you may need a break, and allow one day of indulgence, but remain mindful about what you are eating and really try to enjoy it! After that one day of sheer indulgence, resume your eating/exercise commitment. While you might worry that this will set you back a few hard-fought pounds, it generally does not. It can help you recharge your motivational battery and restart your next four to six weeks of behavior changes to achieve your eventual target. While the example used here focuses on diet, the principle remains true for any long-range goal. Planning for and taking that break helps you to cement your progress and restart your momentum toward your next goal.

## *9. Get some extra help*

Some changes in behavior can be pretty lonely, and you may want to get some outside help and support. It is often easier to change eating patterns if others in your family are doing the same thing. Jogging or walking alone is typically less interesting than when someone else goes with you, especially if they like to chat. Whether you enjoy what they are saying or you have heard those stories before, it distracts you from wondering how far you have walked and how much farther before you are done. One of our patients, a supervisor in a clinical agency, held daily phone meetings with each of her four subordinates to discuss the cases they were handling. She started making these calls from her cell phone using her earphones while she walked. The conversations distracted her and allowed her to squeeze in her weekday exercise while meeting her occupational demands. She liked the fact that she was getting paid to improve her health. And, in her opinion, her ideas actually seemed better during these walks.

Competition may also help. A 66-year-old overweight man told us about his losing 40 pounds in a charity contest at work some years before. He attributed his success to one reason: his coworker lost 39 pounds. He realized just how much he needed someone to beat. But now, in retirement, he did not know what to do with his competitive urges. He needed to find someone new who he could cajole into a weight loss contest. And then, once successful, he would have to develop a different approach to keeping it off. Our response to his plan? "Bet you can't do it."

There are also a number of new approaches made possible by technology that will track your steps when walking; calculate the calories, points, or carbohydrates you eat; measure how many minutes you have used your CPAP each night; and even give you interactive coaching to support the goals you want to achieve. And then there are the "old school" but still valuable support groups, such as WeightWatchers and various 12-step groups. Because people are social animals, they often do better when they can share their goals and approaches with others.

## 10. Don't give up

Most of the failures in long-term behavior change are simply the result of giving up. Something hasn't worked as well as you had hoped or you ran into an injury, a life setback, or some larger problem that has side-tracked you. Fine. That is really okay, so long as it is not permanent. The trick to success in behavior change is to acknowledge that you are off track or stalled, then refocus on your goal without blaming yourself. And then restart.

When our patients wonder "will I ever reach my goal?," we respond with a story based on the nearly disastrous 1970 NASA *Apollo 13* mission to the moon in which almost everything went wrong. Famed for the expression "Houston, we have a problem," the three-member flight crew and dozens of engineers on the ground had to improvise ways to conserve power, modify the air system, and repurpose material after the onboard computers failed and fuel tanks exploded. The 1995 movie about this mission has a great scene in which Jim Lovell, the pilot, played by Tom Hanks, has no onboard computer to plot a reentry path. He scribbles hand calculations to determine how the crew can safely enter Earth's atmosphere, threading a needle between a fiery too-vertical descent and a too-shallow trajectory that will bounce them off the atmosphere into deep space. When he expresses his anxiety about the outcome, the Mission Control flight director gives him the best advice: he instructs everyone to just "work the problem."

While most of our behavior change problems are much less intense, the advice remains the same: work the problem. Stop wondering what might happen. Stop assigning blame, either to others or yourself. Avoid the mental traps that take up time and emotional space. If something did not work as planned, there is probably a discoverable reason. When you begin to lose faith, it is time to reexamine your roadblocks, reformulate your approach, figure out what steps to take, and begin again.

———

In the next and final chapter, we will attack some common problems by applying elements of this 10-step approach.

CHAPTER 14

# Applying the Change
# Formula to Your Life

---

Now let's apply the change formula to three specific behaviors: smoking cessation, CPAP use, and exercise. Each of these plays a critical role in dementia prevention and provides opportunities for successful change.

## Smoking Cessation

Cigarettes have been part of the public health discussion for years. In the 1930s and 1940s, cigarettes were widely advertised in print, radio, and television media. Some even featured doctor-based brand endorsements. A 1930 Lucky Strike magazine advertisement claimed that "20,679 physicians say 'Luckies are less irritating.'" In 1946, a Philip Morris ad boasted, "More doctors smoke Camels than any other cigarette." Tobacco manufacturers, although secretly recognizing that smoking was unhealthy, suggested that health professionals endorsed their brand, a convincing argument that smoking was safe or that the pleasure of smoking outweighed the risks.

These claims, along with cigarette brand advertising, came to an end with the growing realization that all cigarettes are extremely unhealthy and smoking creates an enormous cost to society. Today's warning labels on cigarette packs, mandated public health warnings, minimum purchasing ages, locational restrictions, and high taxes discourage consumption and generate revenue for health care. Today, many insurance companies and the businesses that provide health insurance to their employees sponsor programs to help people quit. While there has been a 20 percent reduction in smokers just since 2005, current CDC statistics reported that there are still 34 million Americans who continue to smoke (not to mention the many more smokers in other countries where people often begin at younger ages). One in five deaths in this country are attributed to smoking, and smokers die, on average, 10 years earlier than those who do not smoke.

As you read previously, cigarette smoking is directly and indirectly linked to dementia. If you are a smoker, this is just one more reason not to smoke. Probably you would rather not be a smoker. The CDC points out that 68 percent of those polled in 2015 wanted to stop and half of all smokers had made an attempt to stop smoking in the previous year. Sadly, they report that only 7.5 percent of those who attempt to quit succeed. Clinically, we encounter few people who want to continue smoking. They are typically elderly, with 50- to 60-year smoking histories and advanced respiratory illness but who feel that they do not have many pleasures left in their lives and that it is too late for them to change. They recognize but minimize their health problems that are due to their smoking. They complain that they do not have enough places to smoke and that cigarettes are too expensive. For the rest of us who are currently smokers, the question is not whether to smoke but how to stop.

There have been many approaches to smoking cessation, including medications (Chantix, Wellbutrin, Zyban) to reduce the urge, nicotine replacement (patch, gum, electronic cigarettes), publication of public health tips, hypnosis, and psychotherapy. All of these work for some people and for some periods of time. You may have tried some or all. But, if you still smoke, the behavioral change steps outlined in the previous chapter may give you some new tools.

## 1. Identify an area for change and reframe it

You want to reduce and eliminate your tobacco smoking. You recognize that smoking increases your risk for cancer and heart disease, high blood pressure, and breathing problems. You have heard that you may not live as long. You experience a loss of smell and taste. You cannot run, play ball, or lift up a child without coughing or gasping for air. You can do the math and see that smoking one pack of cigarettes per day could be costing you 3,500 dollars per year. You recognize that it interrupts your ability to sit through a movie or TV show. And now, you also see that smoking increases your dementia risk.

As a first step, you should become *mindful* or aware of your smoking patterns. To counteract the automatic nature of this habit, we invite you to count exactly how many cigarettes you smoke every day, pay attention to when you smoke, and identify the situations when you smoke. Think of what you are doing right before you light up—what triggers you to reach for a cigarette? Is part of it physiological, a craving your body feels in response to a drop in the nicotine levels within your brain? Or do you smoke out of habit, to participate in a social ritual, or in response to stress or boredom? Have your cigarettes become your buddies for a car ride, while talking on the phone, or while watching TV? Do you smoke right after meals or snacks? Do you smoke as preparation before potentially stressful meetings or encounters? How many cigarettes do you smoke even when you don't really want to? How many cigarettes do you leave, burning in the ashtray, because you lit them without really thinking?

By reviewing your habits and patterns you will discover that smoking is a very complex set of behaviors and that you probably smoke for different reasons at different times. Understanding this complexity is very important and can help you to develop different strategies for different situations. One size does not fit all, and just saying "no" is probably not enough. You need to be more creative. You may choose to set up a barrier to inhibit automatic smoking (wrapping your pack in rubber bands that must be undone) or entertaining yourself with a game on your phone instead of smoking when you are bored. Keeping your hands busy by knitting or crocheting might keep you from having a cigarette. You might limit your smoking to only outside the house or only in the afternoon.

We also suggest that you rethink or reframe the concept of quitting. How you think about this change in your behavior may impact your success. Nobody wants to be a quitter. It sounds like you are giving up something valuable or failing at something you could not master. You want to be a winner. Ask yourself, "How would I feel by beating a terrible habit? What can I gain?" Imagine next year this time, looking back and seeing yourself as a former smoker. Develop a mental picture of walking up a flight of stairs without huffing and puffing. See yourself sitting through a movie without needing a smoking break. Fantasize about smelling fresh flowers, enjoying the subtle flavors of food or a glass of wine, or kissing someone with fresh breath. Calculate how much money you could save and use those savings to buy holiday presents or take a vacation. Reframing the problem prepares you to take the next step.

## 2. Set specific goals

Please do not say that you will "try" to quit. Think about Yoda! Your goal is not to try, but to do, to accomplish, to succeed. You must start by setting specific, measurable, and reasonable goals. You cannot be vague.

You need to count how many cigarettes you smoke, when you smoke, and where you smoke so that your goals are clear and quantifiable.

For example, suppose that you smoke one pack (20 cigarettes) per day and that you smoke in your house, where you also work. You have your first cigarette when you wake up, another with coffee each morning, one after lunch and dinner, and the others scattered throughout the day and evening. You also smoke when you drink a cocktail or beer and while you drive. If this is you, you live in a target-rich environment for smoking, with very few off-limits places, a number of triggers to smoke, and flexibility as to when you smoke. Your first job is to reduce the scope of these smoking opportunities, creating smoking-free times, places, or situations.

## 3. Expect and foresee obstacles

Before we get too far, we need to identify what can go wrong. It is highly likely that you have tried to stop smoking in the past but eventually returned, either immediately, after a few weeks, or even months or years later. Statistics tell us that 9 of 10 people do return to smoking. By analyzing those returns to smoking, you may be able to foresee potholes on the road before you fall into them.

Let's imagine that you threw away your cigarettes on one national Great American Smokeout Day. You felt strong and great. Or maybe you felt "flu-like" for a day or two. This is not unusual. And then you were back to smoking a week later. What happened? That becomes the question for you to examine. Was it a disappointment in a relationship? Someone offered you a cigarette and you thought "how could one hurt?" Did you encounter an emotional situation that you had not anticipated? Did you need a smoke to calm down, to celebrate, or simply take a break? Did you keep a backup pack in a desk drawer, which kept screaming "smoke me!"

These obstacles, once understood, can lead to more successful approaches. You may realize that disappointment hurts but does not require nicotine, nor will smoking repair the relationship or the feelings of loss. You may become aware that other people trigger your urge to smoke and that you have to strategize how to stay away from them at vulnerable times. Maybe you need to take your work break inside rather than outside in the designated smoking area where you will feel deprived or someone may offer you a smoke. Maybe you should drink coffee where you cannot smoke because these two habits have become so intertwined. Maybe you recognize an uncomfortable fact, that you are a "smoke-aholic," physiologically vulnerable to nicotine, a highly addictive substance. So "just one" is the start of your next pack. Knowing yourself and your habits gives you ammunition to change or develop alternative approaches.

## 4. *Examine your* buts

Frequently we see people who know that they *should* quit *but* they cannot imagine doing it forever. They believe that giving up cigarettes will have to be permanent. And since any permanent decision is irrevocable, they believe that they must find the "perfect time" to stop, a time when nothing emotionally difficult is on the horizon or when there are no joyful occasions to celebrate with a cigarette. Since this perfect time cannot be imagined—they will almost certainly face something emotional in the future—they decide to wait for a "better" time.

This "perfect time" *but* will scuttle almost anyone. Life is full of stresses as well as celebrations. It also makes an irrational assumption that you are locked permanently into any decision that you make. In reality, life's highway has a lot of off ramps and even turnarounds you can take. It also projects well too far into the future. We live today, hour by hour and minute by minute. It really is one day at a time.

Whatever your *but* looks like, we suggest that you examine it, get familiar with it, say it out loud or write it down. Tell someone else about it. See what they think. Then see what you think. Really examine your *but*. Does it make sense to you? Do you have to live your life listening to it? In many cases, when you examine your objection critically, you conclude that you should lead with your head, not your *but*.

## 5. Take baby steps

The baby step is to focus on the present and make small changes. Start by delaying your next cigarette. Put it off for an hour. See how you feel then. Procrastinate for another hour. Do something else in the meantime. If it is late at night, go to bed instead. If it is daytime, take a walk. Hours can turn into days, and days can be strung together. After a while without smoking, cigarettes will very likely become less important to you. One day you will wonder why you ever smoked. Each day without smoking is better than a day when you do smoke. Baby steps.

## 6. Use the just-noticeable difference, or JND

This is a very controversial approach we have been using with confirmed smokers who are being pressured to quit by others or who don't believe that they can ever not smoke. As far as we know, there are no studies showing that it works. But it might work for you because your initial buy-in is so painless. It's all about the JND. Suppose you smoke a pack every day, 20 cigarettes in total. We recommend that you continue to smoke 20 cigarettes every day for the next week. Not difficult, is it? You have not had to change anything. The following week, we *want* you to smoke 19 cigarettes each day. No more, no less. Also, not difficult. You recognize that 19 versus 20 is undetectable. It is below your JND. In week three, you smoke 18 cigarettes every day. Again, no big deal because you were smoking 19 before. But now you are counting your cigarettes and slowly paying more attention to when you smoke and why you smoke. You discover that you are not missing anything by smoking 18 per day. In fact, you have been putting the extras aside and, by the end of week four, at 17 cigarettes per day, you have saved two extra packs that you did not have to buy. That could be a 20 dollar bill. Take a 20 dollar bill out of your wallet and put it in a safe place.

So, you keep on going, one less cigarette per day each week and see how far you can go. Can you get to 10 cigarettes? How about 5? If you feel uncomfortable taking the next step, stop where you are and stay there for a while. You are not in a hurry. After smoking for years, you can quit at a pace that works for you.

This approach relies on the reduction each week being so minimal, in comparison to the previous week's consumption, that you avoid feeling deprived and you begin to acquire mastery of your habit. Each reduction is below your JND.

## 7. Play it where it lays

Throughout this process you should focus on where you are and not where you think you should be. All progress is good. Please avoid blaming yourself for not having done this before. You are where you are. It is what it is. When you wonder, "Why didn't I do this years ago?" the correct answer is, "Because I didn't." And isn't it good that you did not wait longer?

## 8. The rest stop: Take a break and check out your surroundings

A break is a time to take stock, not a decision to resume smoking. Because nicotine is addictive, you may need to label yourself as a "smoke-aholic" who cannot have "just one." This is not like a low-carbohydrate diet that allows you to have a carb "blow-out day" after a month or two of successful dieting. Nicotine is a drug and, over the course of many years of smoking, it has carved out millions of nicotinic receptor sites in your brain cells, just waiting to be stimulated again.

Now is the time to consider what is working, what can be improved, and where you have had problems that can be fixed. While you can take some credit for your progress, you will not be out of the woods. Don't become that football player who begins the touchdown dance on the five-yard line, only to have the ball stripped from behind. Crossing this goal line of smoking cessation is just one play, not the end of the game. There are many more games on your schedule.

## 9. Get some extra help

You may benefit from coaching, hypnosis, nicotine gum, nicotine patches, or pharmaceuticals such as bupropion (Zyban or Wellbutrin) and Chantix. These smoking cessation aids add weapons to your arsenal in the battle against cigarettes, and we want you to have every advantage. Talk to your doctor, your therapist, your friends, and family, especially if they have been successful. They may have some tips, and they will almost always give you support.

## 10. Don't give up

Perhaps the most important advice is to persevere. The National Epidemiologic Survey on Alcohol and Related Conditions (NESARC) in 2013 found a nearly 50 percent smoking relapse rate even after a full year of abstinence, with more than a third of people returning to cigarettes after two years. Even after five years, one in four people go back to smoking. This is a long-haul process. Don't give up.

# CPAP Success

According to published figures, one in seven people ages 30 to 69, representing nearly a billion people worldwide, suffers from obstructive sleep apnea (OSA). And almost half of these people have moderate to severe OSA, failing to breathe properly more than 15 times per hour while they sleep. This amounts to 24 million people in the United States, second only to China in prevalence. The true numbers are likely higher, since OSA is three times more probable if you are over age 70, an age group not covered in the estimate. As we discussed in previous chapters, sleep apnea is associated with a host of dementia-creating conditions, including hypoxemia (inadequate oxygen in your blood) leading to hypoxia (inadequate oxygen in your tissues), diabetes, hypertension, stroke, heart attack, atrial fibrillation, and depression. Apnea also interferes with weight loss, energy, and sexual function. As you saw in chapter 6, oxygen is a really important thing.

## 1. Identify an area for change

Sleeping is *not* the area for change. Many people with OSA believe that they sleep well, despite having multiple "mini-arousals" of partial awakening of which they are unaware. In fact, people with apnea often fall asleep quite easily in bed, as well as in their easy chair, the couch, a theater seat, and even the driver's seat of their car. The problem is that they are not *breathing* while sleeping. The obstruction in their airway, caused by age, obesity, or having a crowded and narrow airway, has cut off the air getting to their lungs. And, at more than five times per hour, this reduction or stoppage in breathing means that the red blood cells cannot get oxygen from the air and carry it through the blood vessels to your brain, heart, and other essential organs.

To repeat ourselves from earlier chapters, common symptoms of sleep apnea include too-rapid sleep onset, loud snoring, gasping for breaths and flailing around, waking up to urinate several times each night, having morning headaches, feeling tired even after sleeping, being distractible or disorganized, needing to nap, or dozing off when sitting quietly.

## 2. Set specific goals

So, the goal is to breathe while sleeping, to get more air to the lungs by keeping your airway open. And the best way to do that is by putting room air under enough pressure to keep your airway open. Continuous positive airway pressure (CPAP) uses a very sophisticated and quiet machine that pulls in room air through a filter, increases the air pressure, and pushes pressurized air through a flexible tube and into a mask that you wear over your nose or over your nose and mouth. It usually works very effectively, reducing your apneic episodes to normal, but only if you use it.

Unfortunately, treatment for OSA often fails! According to a 2008 review, only 17 to 54 percent of adults with sleep apnea use CPAP, the most successful treatment, consistently and many of them don't use it throughout the night or when they nap.

## 3. Expect and foresee obstacles

Because of this historically high failure rate, you must expect problems. The first hurdle to success is mental. You did not grow up expecting to wear a mask over your face while you sleep. The thought of it can make you feel old, sick, or tethered to a machine. While you may have seen a character in a TV show or in a movie using CPAP, you never imagined being that person. Because you are sleeping, you have not seen yourself flailing around and gasping for air while asleep, although one study using night vision photography found this to be a very motivating factor. You may worry that your bed partner will no longer think of you as sexy, even though the CPAP mask goes on only *after* any amorous activity. If you have been claustrophobic, you may worry that you will experience anxiety or choking, despite research finding just the opposite will occur. You will breathe easier with the mask than you have without it. Maybe you have been so firmly opposed to CPAP that you refuse to get a sleep test. You just don't want to know what the test might show.

If you are reluctant, you have a lot of company. While you may be lucky enough to know someone who uses CPAP and gets great results, the failure rates indicate that you more likely know someone who failed to stick with treatment. In either case, you have the opportunity to make up your own mind.

## 4. *Examine your* buts

Appreciate your objections. You don't want to feel old, sick, or unsexy. You never imagined that this would be you. You would like to breathe whenever you sleep *but* you "cannot imagine" wearing a CPAP mask. So, we suggest that you imagine something else. Use your mind to help you. Imagine being a fighter pilot and strapping on your oxygen mask before you take off in your jet. Imagine putting on a respirator and mask so you can scuba dive and swim with a school of brightly colored fish. Imagine the breeze blowing through your thatched roof hut as you sleep in a tropical paradise. And imagine that you are bathing your brain in oxygen so that it works at top capacity.

Maybe you tried CPAP but gave up. You were diagnosed with OSA, sent home with a CPAP machine after a quick hour of explanation, and could not get comfortable when you put it on. You could not fall asleep or you awakened after a short time and ripped the mask off your face.

We see many people in this situation and encourage them to try again, but this time differently.

## 5. Take baby steps

Here is where we introduce you to CPAP Success, an approach that we developed and have used successfully with many patients. CPAP Success starts with small steps, the first being for you to wear your CPAP mask while you are awake!

We instruct our new CPAP patients to take their mask and disconnect it from the connecting hose. It pops right off. You now have a large opening through which you can breathe easily. We would instruct you to wear your mask by itself for 15 minutes each day for a week while you are awake and doing something pleasant, like listening to music, meditating, watching TV, or just relaxing. While wearing it, you should adjust the straps that hold the mask in place on your face, changing the tightness or looseness of the headgear to find the most comfortable level of pressure on your head and face. We would ask you to put it on and take it off several or more times. We want you to become very comfortable with the feel of the mask, all the while you are awake and comfortable. This first baby step reassures you that you can control the mask feel and fit, all the while breathing easily. If you are claustrophobic, you will really benefit from knowing that you are in control of the mask. You should do this 15-minute exercise every day for an entire week, well before you start to wear it at night.

During the second week, you would do the same thing every day, except now you connect the hose to the mask, attach it to your CPAP machine, fill the water chamber that humidifies the air, and turn on the power. For 15 minutes every day, while you relax, you feel the flow of moisturized air. You continue to practice adjusting the headgear, taking the mask off and putting it back on again. For 15 minutes you learn to breathe normally and appreciate how easy it is to get comfortable. But you are still not using it at night.

By the third week, you are ready to wear your CPAP in bed and when you want to fall asleep. Having succeeded in such a positive two-week training period, you can now put on the mask in bed, turn on the machine, and fall asleep while comfortably wearing your mask. Does this approach work? Most of the time, yes. In fact, we ran two pilot projects in which this approach resulted in 70 percent and 90 percent success (defined by Medicare adherence criteria), even for patients who already had cognitive impairment, diagnosed as mild cognitive impairment or dementia.

## 6. Use the just-noticeable difference, or JND

Most people who use CPAP Success discover that they sleep three to four hours before they awaken, either because they become uncomfortable or because they still have to use the bathroom. Adapting the JND concept to CPAP, we would encourage you to expand your usage time by simply repeating the process. If it worked once, it can work again. After you wake up, you can take off your mask, turn off your CPAP, and get out of bed. You can use the bathroom or do something quietly while staying out of bed for 15 minutes. Then, when you return to bed, you just put the mask back on, turn on the CPAP, and repeat the process. For most people this results in several more hours of sleep, and you will eventually learn to sleep through this first awakening.

## 7. Play it where it lays

Sometimes you get stuck. You are fine for five hours but can't return for the third round of CPAP use. That's fine for now. You are already well ahead of where you started, and it is common for people to plateau in any change process. Avoid feeling that you have failed. You have simply not finished the process—which takes us to the next step.

## 8. The rest stop: Take a break and check out your surroundings

Reassessing the successes and limitations is an important stage toward success. Chances are that some nights have been wonderful while others are more difficult. You may need a different mask because you started with small nasal pillows that slip out when you move. Your mask may irritate the bridge of your nose and you need some cushioning. You may need a larger mask because you are a mouth breather. Your humidification settings may need adjustment because of seasonal room temperature changes. Maybe you fall back to sleep after taking off your mask in a semi-awake state. Even if you get five hours of use, you should reassess and work on extending your use. Research shows that the most benefit for CPAP kicks in at six or more hours of use. So, reassess your situation and try again. Remember that your goal is to use CPAP whenever you are asleep (including naps and vacations). Ask yourself, "how many hours don't I want to breathe?" Our answer is always the same: "none."

## 9. Get some extra help

At this point, if you have a problem, you may want to contact your CPAP vendor or sleep medicine doctor so you can try a different mask, have them make an adjustment to the air pressure or level of humidification, or buy a mouth lubricating product (such as XyliMelts) so that you don't awaken with dry gums and a sore throat. Maybe you want to discuss your CPAP use with a friend or relative who is having a good experience. Or maybe join an online CPAP support group. In rare cases,

CPAP use can arouse unexpected emotions related to negative early-life experience. In that case, your best bet is to contact a psychotherapist.

## 10. Don't give up

With the stakes being so high and oxygen being so important to your brain, we strongly encourage you to stick with it. Unfortunately, you will probably not outgrow your sleep apnea, since aging increases the problem. Weight loss, while helpful, often is not enough unless you lose a lot of weight and you are young. Tonsillectomy can improve a crowded airway but is painful and sometimes dangerous in adults. Reducing alcohol intake can reduce its respiratory suppression effect, but only to a point. We believe that a positive sleep apnea diagnosis remains in effect until proven otherwise. So don't stop CPAP until you are cleared by a sleep medicine doctor.

# Exercise

## 1. Identify an area for change

We always ask our patients about exercise. Many don't make eye contact when they reply. They avert their gaze, respond with a sheepish smile, and hesitate while they construct their response. They eventually admit that they should be doing more. Some adopt a politician's response by telling us that they *have* an exercise bicycle, a gym membership, or a history of previous exercise. Others explain that they hate to exercise because it is boring, they are too busy, or they have a physical restriction. In one way or another, each of them recognizes the importance of exercise and their distance from their On Target goal.

But, because exercise and activity are so important for preventing dementia and maintaining cognitive and emotional health, your brain cannot grant you a "free pass" if you are busy, don't really enjoy it, used to be athletic, or even if you have some physical limitation. Your brain does not care about your excuses. All your brain asks is "are you exercising?" So, let's take a look at how you might answer this question differently.

## 2. Set specific goals

How you set your goal will likely determine your success. Again, "trying" is not succeeding. Let us suggest a specific goal and then tell you why this will work. The goal is this: "Take a brisk 10-minute walk, three times every day." It is a specific goal, with a clear-cut prescription in terms of type, duration, and frequency.

Walking is excellent exercise and is well-suited for people of all ages and fitness levels. You can walk even if you need to use a cane or walker or while leaning on a shopping cart or stroller. A brisk walk is defined as walking faster than a leisurely stroll but not so fast that you cannot talk while walking. It can be done outside or on a treadmill, in a grocery or large discount store, in a mall, at your office or factory, or even back and forth within your house. It can be interspersed with other cardiovascular exercises, such as riding a stationary bicycle or swimming.

Ten minutes of walking is actually just five minutes out and five minutes back. You can get close to this by walking when you might drive to a convenience store or the post office, even parking your car farther away from your destination. Walking instead of driving for daily chores and errands is often what separates those societies where people live longer from those who don't.

Exercise is cumulative. Just as five nickels makes a quarter, three 10-minute walks equals one 30-minute walk. And seven 30-minute walks get you 210 minutes of exercise per week, well within the 150 to 300 minutes of weekly exercise recommended by the World Health

Organization and most health groups. Why does this approach work? Essentially because you can do it.

### 3. Expect and foresee obstacles

You may have set up obstacles to exercise by virtue of overlearned habits. You drive to places that are well within your walking range. Our 70-year-old neighbor drives home in her car, stops at the entrance to her 30-foot driveway and methodically angles her car so she can get close enough to her mailbox that she could open her window and retrieve her mail. She is not unable to walk; we see her walking outside her house, examining her plants and flowers. Maybe she thinks she is being efficient, not realizing that she is depriving herself of at least a few minutes of walking every day. By itself, walking to get her mail would not make a great difference. But it could be combined with other changes that would add up to improve her fitness. We invite you to examine your everyday habits and see how many sedentary habits you can change.

### 4. Examine your buts

Suppose you rationalize "I would like to exercise, *but* I am too busy to invest a half hour, or I would exercise *but* I don't have proper exercise equipment, or I would exercise *but* I can't afford a fitness club." If you look closely at your *buts*, you will discover that a 10-minute walk can fit into your schedule quite easily, requires nothing more than a decent pair of walking shoes, and costs nothing.

You could also counter the "too busy" *but* by multitasking on your walk. Why not carry your cell phone when you walk? You can use headphones and listen to an audio book, learn a second language through a program, clear your mind by listening to music, catch up on the news, or learn something from a podcast while you walk. You could use that time to make a phone call to check in with a friend, say hi to a relative, and improve your social connectivity. Maybe you can use your walk to supervise an employee or check in with your boss.

As our patient said, by reducing your "exercise" *but,* your exercise could reduce your butt!

## 5. Take baby steps

While it would be wonderful if you could train to run a marathon, you are probably not in good enough shape to take such a large initial step. Your history of sedentary behavior has deconditioned you. You should avoid the temptation to make up for lost time and start at too high an exertion level. Today's excessive exercise could lead to tomorrow's orthopedic appointment. Injuring yourself by starting too fast, too long, or too vigorously will undermine the consistency of your exercise approach and defeat your program. You will probably abandon your new exercise habit if you are too tired or injured to sustain it.

## 6. Use the just-noticeable difference, or JND

The JND concept for exercise suggests that you very gradually increase your intensity and frequency by small increments. Walk a *little* faster than before or a *little* longer. After mastering 10 minutes, think 11 or 12, not 15. Again, the principle of multiplication is your friend: exercising at a slightly faster pace for 12.5 minutes, three times per day, will get you an extra 52 minutes per week and get your weekly exercise total to a very nice level of 200.

## 7. Play it where it lays

But maybe you cannot walk for 10 minutes three times a day without feeling really tired or experiencing too much pain. Don't criticize yourself. That will only lead to giving up and abandoning your goal. We want you to respect reality and start where you can. Listen to what your body is telling you. Start by walking for 5 minutes each time. You will still build consistency and stamina over time. And you can then increase to 6 minutes when you can, 7 minutes after that, and eventually to 10 minutes. Be patient and you will ultimately reach your goal.

## 8. The rest stop: Take a break and check out your surroundings

How's it going? What have you learned? By taking inventory every few days or weeks, you can reflect on your progress and adapt your approach. Maybe you have learned that some days are easier than others, that it is better for you to exercise on an empty stomach, or conversely, that you are more successful after a meal. Perhaps you need to vary your surroundings so that you don't get bored. Drive to a park and walk there, or check out the shopping in a neighboring town. Or maybe your daily walks coincide with those of someone you have met along the way and you now have a new social connection. By regularly checking in with yourself, you can adapt to changing weather conditions or to your need for variety. Most successful lifestyle and habit changes require periodic adaptation to improve on your initial approach.

## 9. Get some extra help

Here is where you might discover that you would do better with a different pair of shoes or if you join friends who are also walking regularly. Maybe you enjoy keeping a daily diary of your walks, you are motivated by the step-counting of your pedometer app, or you decide to write down thoughts or reflections as you walk. Maybe you like to check off successful walking days on your calendar. Or perhaps you have a friendly competition with your sibling. Don't feel shy about sharing your new habit with your spouse or a friend. Most of us do better with an occasional attaboy or attagirl.

## 10. Don't give up

As with any change in what we do, success comes from starting the change and keeping up the change. So, start now. Put down this book, put on your shoes, and take a walk right now.

AFTERWORD

# But What about . . . ?

We hope that we have answered many of your questions about dementia prevention and have helped you to identify some problem areas where you can begin to make changes that will keep your brain in good shape for years to come. We have no illusions that our book will make a profound difference in your life, but we believe in baby steps and hope that our ideas can be a starting point in your dementia prevention program.

We are continually amazed by the progress we are seeing in dementia prevention awareness and strategies. We had to update several sections of the book while we were writing it, and we expect to see even more relevant research emerging between when we finished writing and you started reading. So, keep your eyes open for new information from trusted, science-based sources.

You may also have questions that we did not answer as fully as you had hoped. If you have some specific questions and are willing to have your questions and our answers published in a follow-up book or the next edition of *Dementia Prevention*, please send us your questions or ideas to questions@braindoc.com. We will answer as many questions as we can and may ask your permission to publish your question (without identifying information) and our response.

# Acknowledgments

When one decides to write a book, especially one like this, the introspective process focuses unforgiving light into all the shadowy corners and dusty hideaways of the soul, where the rough and tumble detritus of life's preceding seventy years is stashed, smashed down, contained, and carefully sequestered, usually only escaping in anxious, disquieting dreams at three o'clock in the morning.

Then, the new day begins—with the chance to write another page, a new story, a better ending. The grace to embrace forgotten moments, grieve the losses, ask and grant forgiveness, celebrate survival, and most importantly, offer thanks to those who helped fashion you. This is a thank-you note to an incredible number of people.

In no particular order, I am especially grateful to the following for sheltering and feeding me in many cases, for allowing me to share in their lives and their families, and for giving me options: the Fortinis; the Szybistys; the DeGrandes; the Howells, especially Kathy; the Barbutos, especially Rosemarie; the Micacchiones; the Tommarellos, especially Peggy and Richard; Dr. James and Mary Stran Grady; and the Mushalanskys, especially Alberta and Joe. And, last but not least, the Grandeys.

While it takes a village to raise a child, I believe it takes hundreds, if not thousands of dedicated people to produce a doctor. I have been blessed with the following talented and dedicated teachers, institutions, and communities who nurtured my curiosity; harnessed my intellect; helped organize my ADHD/apneic brain; modeled self-discipline, restraint, ethics, and compassion; and generously and patiently gave of themselves and their knowledge:

Eileen Farrell, sixth-grade teacher, St. Paul's Grade School, Jersey City, NJ.

Sr. Kathleen, Sr. Matthew, Sr. James, Sr. John, Sr. Francis, and Sr. Regina, Trinity High School 1965–69, as well as Stephen Balaban, Diane Clement Kemeny, Debbie Conrad Treon, Elizabeth Hauser, Dennis Hood and his family, Michael Menard, and Michael Puican.

Dolores Titler, LPN, and the fourth-floor nursing staff, Holy Spirit Hospital, Camp Hill, PA, 1967–69.

Sr. Margaret Berry, Sr. Jane Scully, Sr. Regina Marie Campbell, Edith Benzinger, PhD, Steve Borecky, PhD, Tracey Smart, DO, as well as Mary Anne Linz, MD, Cathy Holdcroft Cauley, and Candy Biller, Carlow University, 1969–91.

The brilliant and gifted educators at Jefferson Medical College in Philadelphia, PA, and Bruce Bennett, MD, Deanna Blisard, MD, and David M. Schaffzin, MD, 1993–97.

Kim Mohn, MD, my internal medicine residency director, and other fine clinicians who trained me at UPMC Mercy Hospital in Pittsburgh, PA, including Charles "Rusty" Reese, MD, Kenneth Smith, MD, James Withers, MD, and Anthony Pinevich, MD, as well as critical care intensivists David Crippen MD, and Harry Rafkin MD, who fostered my love of critical care and research.

Don West, MD, and Douglas Noordsy, MD, Dartmouth Hitchcock Medical Center, Lebanon NH, and Bradley "Vince" Watts, MD, White River Junction Veteran's Administration Hospital–Department of Psychiatry, 2004–7.

Most of all, I am deeply indebted to all the thousands of patients and their families who have allowed me the privilege of caring for them.

Your contributions to this book are immeasurable, boundless, and precious.

*—EC*

It started as somewhat of a lark, spending four days in Boston at our favorite hotel, earning continuing education credits to attend a relatively unserious Harvard Medical School workshop, *Writing, Publishing, and Social Media for Healthcare Professionals.* There we met Joe Rusko, our editor at Johns Hopkins University Press, and embarked on an additional career direction as we approached age 70. Could Emily and I write a book together? It would either kill us or bring us together. We are still here, thankfully even closer, four years and a pandemic later.

Writing this book has allowed us to weave together diverse threads of our professional and personal lives as scientists, clinicians, public speakers, essayists, and occasionally humorists. It has challenged us to stretch our brains' "neuronal networks." It is not easy to review and synthesize a wealth of scientific information across multiple disciplines, examine it critically, and create a unique conceptual framework for this information. Then we had to explain these complex and subtle ideas in terms that can be understood, appreciated, and applied by people of diverse backgrounds. If anyone has decided to reconsider their health and their brain-behavior decisions after reading *Dementia Prevention*, we will feel that all the time and effort has been well-spent. And we thank every reader for putting up with our maiden effort as authors.

A special thanks to Joe Rusko for his excellent support and to Terri Lee Paulsen, who meticulously read every word as our copy editor. Thanks also to two lifetime friends, Kathy Allamong Jacobs, a three-time author, and Jerry Doctrow, for their guidance and help in making connections.

We hope to write a next book, a companion piece for health care providers to help many more patients prevent dementia and to confidently treat those already with dementia. And there may even be a book or two after that. Who knows? Sometimes new things just get easier when you keep doing them.

—*MC*

# For Further Reading

## Introduction. An Ounce of Prevention

Ehrlich JR, Goldstein J, Swenor BK, Whitson H, Langa KM, Veliz P. Addition of vision impairment to a life-course model of potentially modifiable dementia risk factors in the US. *JAMA Neurol*. 2022 Jun 1;79(6):623–626. doi: 10.1001/jamaneurol.2022.0723. Erratum in: *JAMA Neurol*. 2022 Jun 1;79(6):634. PMID: 35467745; PMCID: PMC9039828.

Livingston G, Huntley J, Sommerlad A, et al. Dementia prevention, intervention, and care: 2020 report of the Lancet Commission. *Lancet*. 2020;396(10248):413–446. doi: 10.1016/S0140-6736(20)30367-6. Epub 2020 Jul 30.

Mace NL, Rabins PV. *The 36-hour day: a family guide to caring for people who have Alzheimer disease and other dementia*. 7th ed. Johns Hopkins University Press; 2021.

Royal Society for Public Health. That age old question: how attitudes to ageing affect our health and wellbeing. https://www.rsph.org.uk/our-work/policy/older-people/that-age-old-question.html. Last accessed July 2, 2022.

Zissimopoulos J, Jacobson M, Chen Y, Borson S. Knowledge and attitudes concerning Aducanumab among older Americans after FDA approval for treatment of Alzheimer disease. *JAMA Netw Open*. 2022;5(2):e2148355. doi: 10.1001/jamanetworkopen.2021.48355

## Chapter 1. What Is Dementia?

Ahmed RM, Paterson RW, Warren JD, et al. Biomarkers in dementia: clinical utility and new directions. *J Neurol Neurosurg Psychiatry*. 2014;85(12):1426–1434. doi: 10.1136/jnnp.2014.307662

Amaducci LA, Rocca WA, Schoenberg BS. Origin of the distinction between Alzheimer's disease and senile dementia: how history can clarify nosology. *Neurology.* 1986;36(11): 1497–1499. doi: 10.1212/wnl.36.11.1497

Arvanitakis Z, Shah RC, Bennett DA. Diagnosis and management of dementia: review. *J Am Med Assoc.* 2019;322(16):1589–1599. doi: 10.1001/jama.2019.4782

Barker WW, Luis CA, Kashuba A, et al. Relative frequencies of Alzheimer disease, Lewy body, vascular and frontotemporal dementia, and hippocampal sclerosis in the State of Florida Brain Bank. *Alzheimer Dis Assoc Disord.* 2002;16(4):203–212. doi: 10.1097/00002093-200210000-00001

Benjamin S, MacGillivray L, Schildkrout B, Cohen-Oram A, Lauterbach MD, Levin LL. Six landmark case reports essential for neuropsychiatric literacy. *J Neuropsychiatry Clin Neurosci.* 2018;30(4):279–290. doi: 10.1176/appi.neuro psych.18020027. Epub 2018 Aug 24.

Blazer DG, Yaffe K, Liverman C, eds. *Cognitive aging: progress in understanding and opportunities for action.* National Academies Press; 2015. doi: 10.17226/21693

Boyle PA, Yu L, Wilson RS, Schneider JA, Bennett DA. Relation of neuropathology with cognitive decline among older persons without dementia. *Front Aging Neurosci.* 2013;9(5):50. doi: 10.3389/fnagi.2013.00050

Clionsky M, Clionsky E. Identifying cognitive impairment in the annual wellness visit: who can you trust? *J Fam Pract,* 2011;60(11):653–659.

Dang, C, Maruff, P. SuperAging: current findings yield future challenge: A response to Rogalski and Goldberg. *Alzheimers Dement (Amst).* 2019;11:562–563. doi: 10.1016/j.dadm.2019.05.004

DeTure MA, Dickson DW. The neuropathological diagnosis of Alzheimer's disease. *Mol Neurodegener.* 2019;14(32). doi: 10.1186/s13024-019-0333-5

Drachman DA. The amyloid hypothesis, time to move on: amyloid is the downstream result, not cause, of Alzheimer's disease. *Alzheimers Dement.* 2014 May;10(3):372–380. doi: 10.1016/j.jalz.2013.11.003

Dubois B, Hampel H, Feldman HH et al. Proceedings of the Meeting of the International Working Group (IWG) and the American Alzheimer's Association on "The preclinical state of AD"; July 23, 2015; Washington DC, USA. Preclinical Alzheimer's disease: Definition, natural history, and diagnostic criteria. *Alzheimers Dement.* 2016;12(3):292–323. doi: 10.1016/j.jalz.2016.02.002

Elahi F, Miller B. A clinicopathological approach to the diagnosis of dementia. *Nat Rev Neurol.* 2017 Aug;13(8):457–476. doi: 10.1038/nrneurol.2017.96

Fox N, Petersen R. The G8 Dementia Research Summit—a starter for eight? *Lancet*. 2013;382(9909):1968–1969. doi: 10.1016/S0140-6736(13)62426–5

Goodman RA, Lochner KA, Thambisetty M, Wingo TS, Posner SF, Ling SM. Prevalence of dementia subtypes in United States Medicare fee-for-service beneficiaries, 2011–2013. *Alzheimers Dement*. 2017 Jan;13(1):28–37. doi: 10.1016/j.jalz .2016.04.002. Epub 2016 May 10.

Graff-Radford J. Vascular cognitive impairment. *Continuum*. 2019 Feb;25(1):147–164. doi: 10.1212/CON.0000000000000684

Hale JM, Schneider DC, Mehta NK, Myrskylä M. Cognitive impairment in the U.S.: lifetime risk, age at onset, and years impaired. *SSM Popul Health*. 2020;11:100577. doi: 10.1016/j.ssmph.2020.100577. Erratum in: *SSM Popul Health*. 2020 Dec 10;12:100715.

Imtiaz B, Tolppanen AM, Kivipelto M, Soininen H. Future directions in Alzheimer's disease from risk factors to prevention. *Biochem Pharmacol*. 2014;88(4):661–670. doi: 10.1016/j.bcp.2014.01.003. Epub 2014 Jan 10.

Kapasi A, DeCarli C, Schneider JA. Impact of multiple pathologies on the threshold for clinically overt dementia. *Acta Neuropathol*. 2017;134(2):171–186. doi: 10.1007/s00401-017-1717-7. Epub 2017 May 9.

Katzman R. The prevalence and malignancy of Alzheimer disease: a major killer. *Alzheimers Dement*. 2008;4(6):378–380. doi: 10.1016/j.jalz.2008.10.003. Epub 2008 Oct 22.

Knopman DS, Petersen RC, Jack CR. A brief history of "Alzheimer disease": multiple meanings separated by a common name. *Neurology*, 2019; 92(22):1053–1059. doi: 10.1212/WNL.0000000000007583

Marin-Oto M., Vicente EE, Marin JM. Long term management of obstructive sleep apnea and its comorbidities. *Multidiscip Respir Med*, 2019;14(1). doi: 10.4081/mrm.2019.24

Meusel L-AC, Greenwood CE, Maione A, Tchistiakova E, MacInstosh BJ, Anderson NC. Cardiovascular risk and encoding-related hippocampal connectivity in older adults. *BMC Neurosci*, 2019;20(37). doi: 10.1186/s12868-019-0518-4

Neumann MA, Cohn R. Incidence of Alzheimer's disease in large mental hospital; relation to senile psychosis and psychosis with cerebral arteriosclerosis. *Arch Neurol Psychiatry*. 1953;69(5):615–636. doi: 10.1001/archneurpsyc .1953.02320290067008

Nowakowski RS. Stable neuron numbers from cradle to grave. *Proc Natl Acad Sci*

*USA.* 2006;103(33):12219–12220. doi: 10.1073/pnas.0605605103. Epub 2006 Aug 7.

Penke B, Szűcs M, Bogár F. Oligomerization and conformational change turn monomeric β-amyloid and tau proteins toxic: their role in Alzheimer's pathogenesis. *Molecules.* 2020; 25. doi: 10.3390/molecules25071659

Rodriguez RD, Grinberg L. Argyrophilic grain disease: an underestimated tauopathy. *Dement Neuropsychol.* 2015;9:2–8. doi: 10.1590/S1980-57642015 DN91000002

Strassnig M, Ganguli M. About a peculiar disease of the cerebral cortex: Alzheimer's original case revisited. *Psychiatry.* 2005;2:30–33.

Volk B. How to keep your brain from shrinking. *Life Extension Magazine.* https://www.lifeextension.com/magazine/2015/2/combat-age-related-brain-atrophy?utm_source=cj.com&utm_medium=affiliate&utm_campaign=5250933&cjevent=37c6e18e850611eb82fa035f0a240613

Wang H, Li T, Barbarino P, et al. Dementia care during COVID-19. *Lancet.* 2020; 395(10231):1190–1191. doi: 10.1016/S0140-6736(20)30755-8. Epub 2020 Mar 30.

Yu J-T, Xu W, Tan C-C, et al. Evidence-based prevention of Alzheimer's disease: systematic review and meta-analysis of 243 observational prospective studies and 153 randomised controlled trials. *J Neurol Neurosurg.* 2020. doi: 10.1136/jnnp-2019-321913

## Chapter 2. Normal Cognitive Aging

Andersen SL. Centenarians as models of resistance and resilience to Alzheimer's disease and related dementias. *Adv Geriatr Med Res.* 2020;2(3):e200018. doi: 10.20900/agmr20200018. Epub 2020 Jul 3.

Boldrini M, Fulmore CA, Tartt AN, et al. Human hippocampal neurogenesis persists throughout aging. *Cell Stem Cell.* 2018;22(4):589–599.e5. doi: 10.1016/j.stem.2018.03.015

Boyle PA, Wilson RS, Yu L, et al. Much of late life cognitive decline is not due to common neurodegenerative pathologies. *Ann Neurol.* 2013;74(3):478–489. doi: 10.1002/ana.23964. Epub 2013 Jul 10.

DeCarli C. Clinically asymptomatic vascular brain injury: a potent cause of cognitive impairment among older individuals. *J Alzheimers Dis.* 2013;33 Suppl 1(0 1):S417–426. doi: 10.3233/JAD-2012-129004

Exalto LG, Quesenberry CP, Barnes D, Kivipelto M, Biessels GJ, Whitmer RA. Midlife risk score for the prediction of dementia four decades later. *Alzheimers Dement.* 2014;10(5):562–570. doi: 10.1016/j.jalz.2013.05.1772. Epub 2013 Sep 10.

Freeze WM, Jacobs HIL, de Jong JJ, et al. White matter hyperintensities mediate the association between blood-brain barrier leakage and information processing speed. *Neurobiol Aging.* 2020;85:113–122. doi: 10.1016/j.neurobiolaging .2019.09.017. Epub 2019 Sep 27.

Harrington KD, Schembri A, Lim YY, et al. Estimates of age-related memory decline are inflated by unrecognized Alzheimer's disease. *Neurobiol Aging.* 2018;70:170–179. doi: 10.1016/j.neurobiolaging.2018.06.005. Epub 2018 Jun 11.

López-Otín C, Blasco MA, Partridge L, Serrano M, Kroemer G. The hallmarks of aging. *Cell.* 2013;153(6):1194–1217. doi: 10.1016/j.cell.2013.05.039

Masur DM, Sliwinski M, Lipton RB, Blau AD, Crystal HA. Neuropsychological prediction of dementia and the absence of dementia in healthy elderly persons. *Neurology.*1994;44:1427–1432.

Parikh NS, Kumar S, Rosenblatt R, et al. Association between liver fibrosis and cognition in a nationally representative sample of older adults. *Eur J Neurol.* 2020;27(10):1895–1903. doi: 10.1111/ene.14384. Epub 2020 Jul 20.

Rogalski EJ. Don't forget—age is a relevant variable in defining SuperAgers. *Alzheimers Dement.* 2019;11:560–561. doi: 10.1016/j.dadm.2019.05.008

Rogalski EJ, Gefen T, Shi J, et al. Youthful memory capacity in old brains: anatomic and genetic clues from the Northwestern SuperAging Project. *J Cogn Neurosci.* 2013;25(1):29–36. doi: 10.1162/jocn_a_00300

Salthouse TA. Decomposing age correlations on neuropsychological and cognitive variables. *J Int Neuropsychol Soc.* 2009;15(5):650–661. doi: 10.1017 /S1355617709990385. Epub 2009 Jul 2.

Seo SW, Gottesman RF, Clark JM, et al. Nonalcoholic fatty liver disease is associated with cognitive function in adults. *Neurology.* 2016;86(12):1136–1142. doi: 10.1212/WNL.0000000000002498. Epub 2016 Feb 24.

Sliwinski M, Lipton RB, Buschke H, Stewart W. The effects of preclinical dementia on estimates of normal cognitive functioning in aging. *J Gerontol.* 1996;51B(4):217–225.

Sorrells SF, Paredes MF, Cebrian-Silla A, et al. Human hippocampal neurogenesis drops sharply in children to undetectable levels in adults. *Nature.* 2018;555(7696):377–381. doi: 10.1038/nature25975. Epub 2018 Mar 7.

Vannini P, d'Oliere Uquillasc F, Jacobs HIL, et al. Decreased meta-memory is associated with early tauopathy in cognitively unimpaired older adults. *Neuroimage Clin.* 2019;24. doi: 10.1016/j.nicl.2019.102097

## Chapter 3. Genetics and Early-Life Factors

Andersen SL. Centenarians as models of resistance and resilience to Alzheimer's disease and related dementias. *Adv Geriatr Med Res.* 2020;2(3):e200018. doi: 10.20900/agmr20200018. Epub 2020 Jul 3.

Arboleda-Velasquez JF, Lopera F, O'Hare M, et al. Resistance to autosomal dominant Alzheimer's disease in an APOE3 Christchurch homozygote: a case report. *Nat Med.* 2019;25(11):1680–1683. doi: 10.1038/s41591-019-0611-3. Epub 2019 Nov 4.

Baker BH, Lugo-Candelas C, Wu H, et al. Association of prenatal acetaminophen exposure measured in meconium with risk of attention-deficit/hyperactivity disorder mediated by frontoparietal network brain connectivity. *JAMA Pediatr.* 2020;174(11):1073–1081. doi: 10.1001/jamapediatrics.2020.3080

Bale TL. Sex matters. *Neuropsychopharmacology.* 2019;44(1):1–3. doi: 10.1038 /s41386-018-0239-x. Epub 2018 Oct 10.

Belloy ME, Napolioni V, Han SS, Le Guen Y, Greicius MD; Alzheimer's Disease Neuroimaging Initiative. Association of Klotho-VS heterozygosity with risk of Alzheimer disease in individuals who carry APOE4. *JAMA Neurol.* 2020;77(7):849–862. doi: 10.1001/jamaneurol.2020.0414

Bove R, Secor E, Chibnik LB, et al. Age at surgical menopause influences cognitive decline and Alzheimer pathology in older women. *Neurology.* 2014;82(3):222–229. doi: 10.1212/WNL.0000000000000033. Epub 2013 Dec 11.

Cairns A, Poulos G, Bogan R. Sex differences in sleep apnea predictors and outcomes from home sleep apnea testing. *Nat Sci Sleep.* 2016;8:197–205. doi: 10.2147/NSS.S101186

Charkoudian N, Hart ECJ, Barnes JN, Joyner MJ. Autonomic control of body temperature and blood pressure: influences of female sex hormones. *Clin Auton Res.* 2017;27(3):149–155. doi: 10.1007/s10286-017-0420-z. Epub 2017 May 9.

Chiò A, Brunetti M, Barberis M, et al. The role of APOE in the occurrence of frontotemporal dementia in amyotrophic lateral sclerosis. *JAMA Neurol.*

2016;73(4):425–430. doi: 10.1001/jamaneurol.2015.4773

Ciudad S, Puig E, Botzanowski T, et al. Aβ(1–42) tetramer and octamer structures reveal edge conductivity pores as a mechanism for membrane damage. *Nature Commun.* 2020;11(1), [3014]. doi: 10.1038/s41467-020-16566-1

Dean DC III, Jerskey BA, Chen K, et al. Brain differences in infants at differential genetic risk for late-onset Alzheimer disease: a cross-sectional imaging study. *JAMA Neurol.* 2014;71(1):11–22. doi: 10.1001/jamaneurol.2013.4544

De Vocht J, Blommaert J, Devrome M, et al. Use of multimodal imaging and clinical biomarkers in presymptomatic carriers of C9orf72 repeat expansion. *JAMA Neurol.* 2020;77(8):1008–1017. doi: 10.1001/jamaneurol.2020.1087

Dominguez JE, Street L, Louis J. Management of obstructive sleep apnea in pregnancy. *Obstet Gynecol Clin North Am.* 2018;45(2):233–247. doi: 10.1016/j.ogc.2018.01.001

Dubal DB, Yokoyama JS. Longevity gene KLOTHO and Alzheimer disease—a better fate for individuals who carry APOE ε4. *JAMA Neurol.* 2020;77(7):798–800. doi: 10.1001/jamaneurol.2020.0112

Fjell AM, Walhovd KB, Fennema-Notestine C, et al. Alzheimer's disease neuroimaging initiative. Brain atrophy in healthy aging is related to CSF levels of Aβ1–42. *Cereb Cortex.* 2010;20(9):2069–2079. doi: 10.1093/cercor/bhp279. Epub 2010 Jan 4.

Foo JN, Chew EGY, Chung SJ, et al. Identification of risk loci for Parkinson disease in Asians and comparison of risk between Asians and Europeans: a genome-wide association study. *JAMA Neurol.* 2020;77(6):746–754. doi: 10.1001/jamaneurol.2020.0428

Goldstein JM, Hale T, Foster SL, Tobet SA, Handa RJ. Sex differences in major depression and comorbidity of cardiometabolic disorders: impact of prenatal stress and immune exposures. *Neuropsychopharmacology.* 2019;44(1):59–70. doi: 10.1038/s41386-018-0146-1. Epub 2018 Jul 7.

Greendale GA, Karlamangla AS, Maki PM. The menopause transition and cognition. *Journal of the American Medical Association.* 2020;323(15):1495–1496. doi: 10.1001/jama.2020.1757

Halsted CH, Wong DH, Peerson JM, et al. Relations of glutamate carboxypeptidase II (GCPII) polymorphisms to folate and homocysteine concentrations and to scores of cognition, anxiety, and depression in a homogeneous Norwegian population: the Hordaland Homocysteine Study. *Am J Clin Nutr.*

2007;86(2):514–521. doi: 10.1093/ajcn/86.2.514

Hamer J, Churchill NW, Hutchison MG, Graham SJ, Schweizer TA. Sex differences in cerebral blood flow associated with a history of concussion. *J Neurotrauma.* 2020;37(10):1197–1203. doi: 10.1089/neu.2019.6800. Epub 2019 Dec 17.

Harshfield GA, Pulliam DA, Alpert BS. Ambulatory blood pressure and renal function in healthy children and adolescents. *Am J Hypertens.* 1994;7(3):282–285. doi: 10.1093/ajh/7.3.282

Ho DSW, Schierding W, Wake M, Saffery R, O'Sullivan J. Machine learning SNP based prediction for precision medicine. *Front Genet.* 2019;10:267. doi: 10.3389 /fgene.2019.00267

Hohman TJ, Kaczorowski CC. Modifiable lifestyle factors in Alzheimer disease: an opportunity to transform the therapeutic landscape through transdisciplinary collaboration. *JAMA Neurol.* 2020;77(10):1207–1209. doi: 10.1001/jamaneurol .2020.1114

Hunt JFV, Vogt NM, Jonaitis EM, et al. Association of neighborhood context, cognitive decline, and cortical change in an unimpaired cohort. *Neurology.* 2021;96(20):e2500–e2512. doi: 10.1212/WNL.0000000000011918. Epub 2021 Apr 14.

Insel PS, Hansson O, Mattsson-Carlgren N. Association between apolipoprotein E ε2 vs ε4, age, and β-amyloid in adults without cognitive impairment. *JAMA Neurol.* 2021;78(2):229–235. doi: 10.1001/jamaneurol.2020.3780

Jara SM, Hopp ML, Weaver EM. Association of continuous positive airway pressure treatment with sexual quality of life in patients with sleep apnea: follow-up study of a randomized clinical trial. *JAMA Otolaryngol Head Neck Surg.* 2018;144(7):587–593. doi: 10.1001/jamaoto.2018.0485

Kaufmann MR, Barth S, Konietzko U, et al. Dysregulation of hypoxia-inducible factor by presenilin/γ-secretase loss-of-function mutations. *Journal of Neurosci.* 2013;33(5):1915–26. doi: 10.1523/JNEUROSCI.3402-12.2013

Kessler RC. Epidemiology of women and depression. *J Affect Disord.* 2003;74(1): 5–13. doi: 10.1016/s0165-0327(02)00426-3

King GD, Chen C, Huang MM, et al. Identification of novel small molecules that elevate Klotho expression. *Biochem J.* 2012;441(1):453–461. doi: 10.1042 /BJ20101909

Kunkle BW, Grenier-Boley B, Sims R, et al. Genetic meta-analysis of diagnosed Alzheimer's disease identifies new risk loci and implicates Aβ, tau, immunity and lipid processing. *Nat Genet.* 2019;51(3):414–430. doi: 10.1038/s41588-019 -0358-2. Epub 2019 Feb 28. Erratum in: *Nat Genet.* 2019 Sep;51(9):1423–1424.

Levine DA, Gross AL, Briceño EM, et al. Association between blood pressure and later-life cognition among black and white individuals. *JAMA Neurol.* 2020;77(7):810–819. doi: 10.1001/jamaneurol.2020.0568

Li H, Wang B, Wang Z, et al. Soluble amyloid precursor protein (APP) regulates transthyretin and Klotho gene expression without rescuing the essential function of APP. *Proc Natl Acad Sci.* 2010;107(40):17362–17367. doi: 10.1073 /pnas.1012568107

Lim YY, Hassenstab J, Goate A, et al. Effect of BDNFVal66Met on disease markers in dominantly inherited Alzheimer's disease. *Ann Neurol.* 2018;84(3):424–435. doi: 10.1002/ana.25299. Epub 2018 Aug 25.

Liu CC, Liu CC, Kanekiyo T, Xu H, Bu G. Apolipoprotein E and Alzheimer disease: risk, mechanisms and therapy. *Nat Rev Neurol.* 2013;9(2):106–118. doi: 10.1038 /nrneurol.2012.263. Epub 2013 Jan 8. Erratum in: *Nat Rev Neurol.* 2013. doi: 10.1038/nmeurol.2013.32. Liu, Chia-Chan [corrected to Liu, Chia-Chen].

Lourida I, Hannon E, Littlejohns TJ, et al. Association of lifestyle and genetic risk with incidence of dementia. *J Am Med Assoc.* 2019;322(5):430–437. doi: 10.1001 /jama.2019.9879

Macey PM, Prasad JP, Ogren JA, et al. Sex-specific hippocampus volume changes in obstructive sleep apnea. *Neuroimage Clin.* 2018;20:305–317. doi: 10.1016 /j.nicl.2018.07.027

Mata IF, Leverenz JB, Weintraub D, et al. APOE, MAPT, and SNCA genes and cognitive performance in Parkinson disease. *JAMA Neurol.* 2014;71(11):1405–1412. doi: 10.1001/jamaneurol.2014.1455

Miller BL. Science denial and COVID conspiracy theories: potential neurological mechanisms and possible responses. *J Am Med Assoc.* 2020;324(22):2255–2256. doi: 10.1001/jama.2020.21332

Miller T, Cudkowicz M, Shaw PJ, et al. Phase 1–2 trial of antisense oligonucleotide tofersen for SOD1 ALS. *N Engl J Med.* 2020;383(2):109–119. doi: 10.1056/NEJM oa2003715

Molloy AM, Pangilinan F, Mills JL, et al. A common polymorphism in HIBCH influences methylmalonic acid concentrations in blood independently of cobalamin. *Am J Hum Genet.* 2016;98(5):869–882. doi: 10.1016/j.ajhg.2016.03.005. Epub 2016 Apr 28.

Montagne A, Nation DA, Sagare AP, et al. APOE4 leads to blood-brain barrier dysfunction predicting cognitive decline. *Nature*. 2020;581(7806):71–76. doi: 10.1038/s41586-020-2247-3. Epub 2020 Apr 29.

Mormino EC, Betensky RA, Hedden T, et al. Amyloid and APOE ε4 interact to influence short-term decline in preclinical Alzheimer disease. *Neurology*. 2014;82(20):1760–1767. doi: 10.1212/WNL.0000000000000431. Epub 2014 Apr 18.

Nordström A, Nordström P. Traumatic brain injury and the risk of dementia diagnosis: a nationwide cohort study. *PLoS Med*. 2018;15(1):e1002496. doi: 10.1371/journal.pmed.1002496

O'Hara R, Luzon A, Hubbard J, Zeitzer JM. Sleep apnea, apolipoprotein epsilon 4 allele, and TBI: mechanism for cognitive dysfunction and development of dementia. *J Rehabil Res Dev*. 2009;46(6):837–850. doi: 10.1682/jrrd.2008.10.0140

Oveisgharan S, Wilson RS, Yu L, Schneider JA, Bennett DA. Association of early-life cognitive enrichment with Alzheimer disease pathological changes and cognitive decline. *JAMA Neurol*. 2020;77(10):1217–1224. doi: 10.1001/jamaneurol.2020.1941

Poewe W, Seppi K, Tanner CM, et al. Parkinson disease. *Nat Rev Dis Primers*. 2017;3:17013. doi: 10.1038/nrdp.2017.13

Proskovec AL, Rezich MT, O'Neill J, et al. Association of epigenetic metrics of biological age with cortical thickness. *JAMA Netw Open*. 2020;3(9):e2015428. doi: 10.1001/jamanetworkopen.2020.15428

Rainville JR, Hodes GE. Inflaming sex differences in mood disorders. *Neuropsychopharmacology*. 2019;44(1):184–199. doi: 10.1038/s41386-018-0124-7. Epub 2018 Jun 19.

Raz L, Knoefel J, Bhaskar K. The neuropathology and cerebrovascular mechanisms of dementia. *J Cereb Blood Flow Metab*. 2016;36(1):172–186. doi: 10.1038/jcbfm.2015.164

Reckelhoff JF. Gender differences in the regulation of blood pressure. *Hypertension*. 2001;37(5):1199–1208. doi: 10.1161/01.hyp.37.5.1199

Reiman EM, Chen K, Alexander GE, et al. Functional brain abnormalities in young adults at genetic risk for late-onset Alzheimer's dementia. *Proc Natl Acad Sci USA*. 2004;101(1):284–289. doi: 10.1073/pnas.2635903100. Epub 2003 Dec 19.

Rosenberg RN, Lambracht-Washington D, Yu G, Xia W. Genomics of Alzheimer disease: a review. *JAMA Neurol.* 2016;73(7):867–874. doi: 10.1001/jamaneurol.2016.0301

Rossor MN, Fox NC, Mummery CJ, Schott JM, Warren JD. The diagnosis of young-onset dementia. *Lancet Neurol.* 2010;9(8):793–806. doi: 10.1016/S1474-4422(10)70159-9

Salihu HM, King L, Patel P, et al. Association between maternal symptoms of sleep disordered breathing and fetal telomere length. *Sleep.* 2015;38(4):559–566. doi: 10.5665/sleep.4570

Salthouse T. Consequences of age-related cognitive declines. *Annu Rev Psychol.* 2012;63:201–226. doi: 10.1146/annurev-psych-120710-100328. Epub 2011 Jul 5.

Schumacher J, Peraza LR, Firbank M, et al. Dysfunctional brain dynamics and their origin in Lewy body dementia. *Brain.* 2019;142(6):1767–1782. doi: 10.1093/brain/awz069

Shively S, Scher AI, Perl DP, Diaz-Arrastia R. Dementia resulting from traumatic brain injury: what is the pathology? *Arch Neurol.* 2012;69(10):1245–1251. doi: 10.1001/archneurol.2011.3747

Sperling RA, Donohue MC, Raman R, et al. Association of factors with elevated amyloid burden in clinically normal older individuals. *JAMA Neurol.* 2020;77(6):735–745. doi: 10.1001/jamaneurol.2020.0387

Spira AP, Blackwell T, Stone KL, et al. Sleep-disordered breathing and cognition in older women. *J Am Geriatr Soc.* 2008;56(1):45–50. doi: 10.1111/j.1532-5415.2007.01506.x. Epub 2007 Nov 28.

Sulzer D, Antonini A, Leta V, et al. COVID-19 and possible links with Parkinson's disease and Parkinsonism: from bench to bedside. *NPJ Parkinsons Dis.* 2020;6:18. doi: 10.1038/s41531-020-00123-0

Sun Y, Fang J, Wan Y, Su P, Tao F. Association of early-life adversity with measures of accelerated biological aging among children in China. *JAMA Netw Open.* 2020;3(9):e2013588. doi: 10.1001/jamanetworkopen.2020.13588

Tanda R, Salsberry PJ, Reagan PB, Fang MZ. The impact of prepregnancy obesity on children's cognitive test scores. *Matern Child Health J.* 2013;17(2):222–229. doi: 10.1007/s10995-012-0964-4

Tshala-Katumbay D, Mwanza JC, Rohlman DS, Maestre G, Oriá RB. A global perspective on the influence of environmental exposures on the nervous system. *Nature.* 2015;527(7578):S187–S192. doi: 10.1038/nature16034

Vo HT, Laszczyk AM, King GD. Klotho, the key to healthy brain aging? *Brain Plast*. 2018;3(2):183–194. doi: 10.3233/BPL-170057

Xu Y, Sun Z. Molecular basis of Klotho: from gene to function in aging. *Endocr Rev*. 2015 Apr;36(2):174–193. doi: 10.1210/er.2013-1079. Epub 2015 Feb 19.

Zhang H, Li Y, Fan Y, et al. Klotho is a target gene of PPAR-gamma. *Kidney Int*. 2008;74(6):732–739. doi: 10.1038/ki.2008.244. Epub 2008 Jun 11.

Zheng H, Koo EH. The amyloid precursor protein: beyond amyloid. *Mol Neurodegener*. 2006;1:5. doi: 10.1186/1750-1326-1-5

Zhou Q, Lin S, Tang R, et al. Role of Fosinopril and Valsartan on Klotho gene expression induced by Angiotensin II in rat renal tubular epithelial cells. *Kidney Blood Press Res*. 2010;33(3):186–192. doi: 10.1159/000316703

## Chapter 4. Midlife Medical Conditions That Affect Dementia Risk

Amarenco P, Kim JS, Labreuche J, et al. A comparison of two LDL cholesterol targets after ischemic stroke. *N Engl J Med*. 2020;382(1):9. doi: 10.1056/NEJM oa1910355. Epub 2019 Nov 18.

Bell RD, Zlokovic BV. Neurovascular mechanisms and blood-brain barrier disorder in Alzheimer's disease. *Acta Neuropathol*. 2009;118(1):103–113. doi: 10.1007 /s00401-009-0522-3. Epub 2009 Mar 25.

Biessels GJ, Whitmer RA. Cognitive dysfunction in diabetes: how to implement emerging guidelines. *Diabetologia*. 2020;63(1):3–9. doi: 10.1007/s00125-019 -04977-9. Epub 2019 Aug 16.

Boehme C, Toell T, Mayer L, et al. The dimension of preventable stroke in a large representative patient cohort. *Neurology*. 2019;93(23):e2121–e2132. doi: 10.1212/WNL.0000000000008573. Epub 2019 Oct 31.

Bonda DJ, Lee HG, Camins A, et al. The critical role of the sirtuin pathway in ageing and Alzheimer disease: mechanistic and therapeutic considerations. *Lancet Neurol*. 2011;10(3):275–279. doi: 10.1016/s1474-4422(11)70013-8

Borland E, Stomrud E, van Westen D, Hansson O, Palmqvist S. The age-related effect on cognitive performance in cognitively healthy elderly is mainly caused by underlying AD pathology or cerebrovascular lesions: implications for cutoffs regarding cognitive impairment. *Alzheimers Res Ther*. 2020;12(1):30. doi: 10.1186/s13195-020-00592-8

Brickman AM, Schupf N, Manly JJ, et al. Brain morphology in older African Americans, Caribbean Hispanics, and whites from northern Manhattan. *Arch Neurol.* 2008;65(8):1053–1061. doi: 10.1001/archneur.65.8.1053

Crane PK, Walker R, Hubbard RA, et al. Glucose levels and risk of dementia. *N Engl J Med.* 2013;369(6):540–548. doi: 10.1056/NEJMoa1215740. Erratum in: *N Engl J Med.* 2013 Oct 10;369(15):1476.

Caunca MR, Simonetto M, Cheung YK, et al. Diastolic blood pressure is associated with regional white matter lesion load: the Northern Manhattan Study. *Stroke.* 2020;51(2):372–378. doi: 10.1161/STROKEAHA.119.025139. Epub 2020 Jan 8.

DeCarli C. Clinically asymptomatic vascular brain injury: a potent cause of cognitive impairment among older individuals. *J Alzheimers Dis.* 2013;33 Suppl 1(01):S417–S426. doi: 10.3233/JAD-2012-129004

Denver P, McClean PL. Distinguishing normal brain aging from the development of Alzheimer's disease: inflammation, insulin signaling and cognition. *Neural Regen Res.* 2018;13(10):1719–1730. doi: 10.4103/1673-5374.238608

Flint AC, Conell C, Ren X, et al. Effect of systolic and diastolic blood pressure on cardiovascular outcomes. *N Engl J Med.* 2019;381(3):243–251. doi: 10.1056/NEJMoa1803180

Gorelick PB, Nyenhuis D. Stroke and cognitive decline. *J Am Med Assoc.* 2015;314(1):29–30. doi: 10.1001/jama.2015.7149

Goss AM, Gower B, Soleymani T, et al. Effects of weight loss during a very low carbohydrate diet on specific adipose tissue depots and insulin sensitivity in older adults with obesity: a randomized clinical trial. *Nutr Metab.* 2020;7(64) doi: 10.1186/s12986-020-00481-9

Graff-Radford J. Vascular cognitive impairment. *Continuum.* 2019;25(1):147–164. doi: 10.1212/CON.0000000000000684

Grinberg LT, Thal DR. Vascular pathology in the aged human brain. *Acta Neuropatholog.* 2010;119(3):277–290. doi: 10.1007/s00401-010-0652-7. Epub 2010 Feb 14.

Grundy SM, Stone NJ, Bailey AL, et al. 2018 AHA/ACC/AACVPR/AAPA/ABC/ACPM/ADA/AGS/APhA/ASPC/NLA/PCNA Guideline on the management of blood cholesterol: a report of the American College of Cardiology/American Heart Association Task Force on Clinical Practice Guidelines. *Circulation.* 2019;139(25):e1082–e1143. doi: 10.1161/CIR.0000000000000625. Epub 2018 Nov 10. Erratum in: *Circulation.* 2019 Jun 18;139(25):e1182–e1186.

Hainsworth AH. White matter lesions in cerebral small vessel disease: Underperfusion or leaky vessels? *Neurology*. 2019;92(15):687–688. doi: 10.1212 /WNL.0000000000007258. Epub 2019 Mar 13.

Huang PL. A comprehensive definition for metabolic syndrome. *Dis Model Mech*. 2009;2(5–6):231–237. doi: 10.1242/dmm.001180

Hughes D, Judge C, Murphy R, et al. Association of blood pressure lowering with incident dementia or cognitive impairment: a systematic review and meta-analysis. *J Am Med Assoc*. 2020;323(19):1934–1944. doi: 10.1001 /jama.2020.4249

Iadecola C. The overlap between neurodegenerative and vascular factors in the pathogenesis of dementia. *Acta Neuropatholog*. 2010;120(3):287–296. doi: 10.1007/s00401-010-0718-6. Epub 2010 Jul 11.

Jellinger KA. Pathology and pathogenesis of vascular cognitive impairment-a critical update. *Front Aging Neurosci*. 2013;5:17. doi: 10.3389/fnagi.2013.00017

Kalaria RN, Akinyemi R, Ihara M. Stroke injury, cognitive impairment and vascular dementia. *Biochimica et Biophysica Acta*. 2016;1862(5):915–925. doi: 10.1016/j.bbadis.2016.01.015. Epub 2016 Jan 22.

Koike MA, Green KN, Blurton-Jones M, Laferla FM. Oligemic hypoperfusion differentially affects tau and amyloid-{beta}. *Am J Pathol*. 2010;177(1):300–310. doi: 10.2353/ajpath.2010.090750. Epub 2010 May 14.

Kuehn BM. In Alzheimer research, glucose metabolism moves to center stage. *J Am Med Assoc*. 2020;323(4):297–299. doi: 10.1001/jama.2019.20939

Lane CA, Barnes J, Nicholas JM, et al. Associations between vascular risk across adulthood and brain pathology in late life: evidence from a British birth cohort. *JAMA Neurol*. 2020;77(2):175–183. doi: 10.1001/jamaneurol.2019.3774.

Lee ATC, Richards M, Chan WC, Chiu HFK, Lee RSY, Lam LCW. Higher dementia incidence in older adults with type 2 diabetes and large reduction in HbA1c. *Age Ageing*. 2019;48(6):838–844. doi: 10.1093/ageing/afz108

Levine DA, Galecki AT, Langa KM, et al. Trajectory of cognitive decline after incident stroke. *J Am Med Assoc*. 2015;314(1):41–51. doi: 10.1001/jama.2015.6968

Lo JW, Crawford JD, Samaras K, et al. Association of prediabetes and type 2 diabetes with cognitive function after stroke: a STROKOG collaboration study. *Stroke*. 2020;51(6):1640–1646. doi: 10.1161/STROKEAHA.119.028428. Epub 2020 May 14.

McAllister TW. Neurobehavioral sequelae of traumatic brain injury: evaluation

and management. *World Psychiatry*. 2008;7(1):3–10. doi: 10.1002/j.2051
-5545.2008.tb00139.x

McMillan JM, Mele BS, Hogan DB, Leung AA. Impact of pharmacological
treatment of diabetes mellitus on dementia risk: systematic review and meta-
analysis. *BMJ Open Diabetes Res Care*. 2018;6(1):e000563. doi: 10.1136/bmjdrc
-2018-000563

Meusel LA-C, Greenwood CE, Maione A, Tchistiakova E, MacIntosh BJ, Anderson ND. Cardiovascular risk and encoding-related hippocampal connectivity in
older adults. *BMC Neurosci*. 2019;20,37. doi: 10.1186/s12868-019-0518-4

Qiu L, Ng G, Tan EK, Liao P, Kandiah N, Zeng L. Chronic cerebral hypoperfusion
enhances tau hyperphosphorylation and reduces autophagy in Alzheimer's
disease mice. *Sci Rep*. 2016 Apr 6;6:23964. doi: 10.1038/srep23964

Román GC. Vascular dementia may be the most common form of dementia in the
elderly. *J Neurolog Sci*. 2002;203–204:7–10. doi: 10.1016/s0022-510x(02)00252-6

Sila CA. Cognitive impairment in chronic heart failure. *Cleve Clin J Med*. 2007;74
Suppl 1:S132–S137. doi: 10.3949/ccjm.74.suppl_1.s132

Smith EE, O'Donnell M, Dagenais G, et al. Early cerebral small vessel disease and
brain volume, cognition, and gait. *Ann Neurol*. 2015;77:251–261. doi: 10.1002
/ana.24320

Sperling RA, Donohue MC, Raman R, et al. Association of factors with elevated amyloid burden in clinically normal older individuals. *JAMA Neurol*.
2020;77(6):735–745. doi: 10.1001/jamaneurol.2020.0387

Tatemichi TK, Paik M, Bagiella E, et al. Risk of dementia after stroke in a hospital-
ized cohort: results of a longitudinal study. *Neurology*. 1994;44(10):1885–1891.
doi: 10.1212/wnl.44.10.1885

Wium-Andersen IK, Osler M, Jørgensen MB, Rungby J, Wium-Andersen MK.
Antidiabetic medication and risk of dementia in patients with type 2 diabetes: a nested case-control study. *Eur J Endocrinol*. 2019;181(5):499–507.
doi: 10.1530/EJE-19-0259

Wolters FJ, Ikram MA. Epidemiology of vascular dementia. *Arterioscler Thromb
Vasc Biol*. 2019;39(8):1542–1549. doi: 10.1161/ATVBAHA.119.311908. Epub 2019
Jul 11.

Xie W, Zheng F, Yan L, Zhong B. Cognitive decline before and after incident coronary events. *J Am Coll Cardiol*. 2019;73(24):3041–3050. doi: 10.1016/j.jacc.2019
.04.019. Erratum in: *J Am Coll Cardiol*. 2019 Sep 3;74(9):1274.

Yang T, Sun Y, Lu Z, Leak RK, Zhang F. The impact of cerebrovascular aging on vascular cognitive impairment and dementia. *Ageing Res Rev*. 2017;34:15–29. doi: 10.1016/j.arr.2016.09.007. Epub 2016 Sep 28.

Zhang J, Chen C, Hua S, et al. An updated meta-analysis of cohort studies: diabetes and risk of Alzheimer's disease. *Diabetes Res Clin Pract*. 2017;124:41–47. doi: 10.1016/j.diabres.2016.10.024. Epub 2016 Nov 9.

Zuccalà G, Cattel C, Manes-Gravina E, Di Niro MG, Cocchi A, Bernabei R. Left ventricular dysfunction: a clue to cognitive impairment in older patients with heart failure. *J Neurol Neurosurg Psychiatry*. 1997;63(4):509–512. doi: 10.1136/jnnp.63.4.509

## Chapter 5. Lifestyle Factors of Smoking, Diet, and Exercise

Abbott RD, White LR, Ross GW, Masaki KH, Curb JD, Petrovitch H. Walking and dementia in physically capable elderly men. *J Am Med Assoc*. 2004;292(12):1447–1453. doi: 10.1001/jama.292.12.1447

Amen DG, Wu J, George N, Newberg A. Patterns of regional cerebral blood flow as a function of obesity in adults. *J Alzheimers Dis*. 2020;77(3):1331–1337. doi: 10.3233/JAD-200655

Baker LD, Frank LL, Foster-Schubert K, et al. Effects of aerobic exercise on mild cognitive impairment: a controlled trial. *Arch Neurol*. 2010;67(1):71–79. doi: 10.1001/archneurol.2009.307

Burns JM, Cronk BB, Anderson HS, et al. Cardiorespiratory fitness and brain atrophy in early Alzheimer disease. *Neurology*. 2008;71(3):210–216. doi: 10.1212/01.wnl.0000317094.86209.cb

Carter S, Clifton PM, Keogh JB. Effect of intermittent compared with continuous energy restricted diet on glycemic control in patients with type 2 diabetes: a randomized noninferiority trial. *JAMA Netw Open*. 2018;1(3):e180756. doi: 10.1001/jamanetworkopen.2018.0756

Chen X, Wang R, Lutsey PL, et al. Racial/ethnic differences in the associations between obesity measures and severity of sleep-disordered breathing: the Multi-Ethnic Study of Atherosclerosis. *Sleep Med*. 2016;26:46–53. doi: 10.1016/j.sleep.2015.06.003. Epub 2015 Jun 25.

Defina LF, Willis BL, Radford NB, et al. The association between midlife cardiorespiratory fitness levels and later-life dementia: a cohort study. *Ann Intern Med*.

2013;158(3):162–168. doi: 10.7326/0003-4819-158-3-201302050-00005

De la Rosa A, Solana E, Corpas R, et al. Long-term exercise training improves memory in middle-aged men and modulates peripheral levels of BDNF and Cathepsin B. *Sci Rep.* 2019;9(1):3337. doi: 10.1038/s41598-019-40040-8

Dhana K, Evans DA, Rajan KB, Bennett DA, Morris MC. Healthy lifestyle and the risk of Alzheimer dementia: Findings from 2 longitudinal studies. *Neurology.* 2020;95(4):e374–e383. doi: 10.1212/WNL.0000000000009816. Epub 2020 Jun 17.

Dolcini J, Wu H, Nwanaji-Enwerem JC, et al. Mitochondria and aging in older individuals: an analysis of DNA methylation age metrics, leukocyte telomere length, and mitochondrial DNA copy number in the VA normative aging study. *Aging.* 2020;12(3):2070–2083. doi: 10.18632/aging.102722. Epub 2020 Feb 2.

Durazzo TC, Mattsson N, Weiner MW; Alzheimer's Disease Neuroimaging Initiative. Smoking and increased Alzheimer's disease risk: a review of potential mechanisms. *Alzheimers Dement.* 2014;10(3 Suppl):S122–S145. doi: 10.1016/j.jalz.2014.04.009

Erickson KI, Voss MW, Prakash RS, et al. Exercise training increases size of hippocampus and improves memory. *Proc Natl Acad Sci USA.* 2011;108(7):3017–3022. doi: 10.1073/pnas.1015950108. Epub 2011 Jan 31.

Frisardi V, Solfrizzi V, Seripa D, et al. Metabolic-cognitive syndrome: a crosstalk between metabolic syndrome and Alzheimer's disease. *Ageing Res Rev.* 2010;9(4):399–417. doi: 10.1016/j.arr.2010.04.007. Epub 2010 May 2.

Grammatikopoulou MG, Goulis DG, Gkiouras K, et al. To keto or not to keto? a systematic review of randomized controlled trials assessing the effects of ketogenic therapy on Alzheimer disease. *Adv Nutr.* 2020;11(6):1583–1602. doi: 10.1093/advances/nmaa073

Guijas C, Montenegro-Burke JR, Cintron-Colon R, et al. Metabolic adaptation to calorie restriction. *Sci Signal.* 2020;13(648):eabb2490. doi: 10.1126/scisignal.abb2490

Hall JR, Wiechmann AR, Johnson LA, et al. Total cholesterol and neuropsychiatric symptoms in Alzheimer's disease: the impact of total cholesterol level and gender. *Dement Geriatr Cogn Disord.* 2014;38(5–6):300–309. doi: 10.1159/000361043. Epub 2014 Jul 4.

Hughes KC, Gao X, Molsberry S, Valeri L, Schwarzschild MA, Ascherio A. Physical activity and prodromal features of Parkinson disease. *Neurology.*

2019;93(23):e2157–e2169. doi: 10.1212/WNL.0000000000008567. Epub 2019 Nov 12.

Ismail Z, Agüera-Ortiz L, Brodaty H, et al. The Mild Behavioral Impairment Checklist (MBI-C): a rating scale for neuropsychiatric symptoms in pre-dementia populations. *J Alzheimers Dis.* 2017;56(3):929–938. doi: 10.3233/JAD-160979

Kimura N, Aso Y, Yabuuchi K, et al. Modifiable lifestyle factors and cognitive function in older people: a cross-sectional observational study. *Front Neurol.* 2019;10:401. doi: 10.3389/fneur.2019.00401

Larson EB, Wang L, Bowen JD, et al. Exercise is associated with reduced risk for incident dementia among persons 65 years of age and older. *Ann Intern Med.* 2006;144(2):73–81. doi: 10.7326/0003-4819-144-2-200601170-00004

Masuki S, Morikawa M, Nose H. High-intensity walking time is a key determinant to increase physical fitness and improve health outcomes after interval walking training in middle-aged and older people. *Mayo Clin Proc.* 2019;94(12):2415–2426. doi: 10.1016/j.mayocp.2019.04.039. Epub 2019 Aug 30.

Morris MC, Tangney CC, Wang Y, Sacks FM, Bennett DA, Aggarwal NT. MIND diet associated with reduced incidence of Alzheimer's disease. *Alzheimer Dement.* 2015;11(9):1007–1014. doi: 10.1016/j.jalz.2014.11.009. Epub 2015 Feb 11.

Moser DA, Doucet GE, Ing A, et al. An integrated brain-behavior model for working memory. *Mol Psychiatry.* 2018;23(10):1974–1980. doi: 10.1038/mp.2017.247. Epub 2017 Dec 5.

Najar J, Östling S, Gudmundsson P, et al. Cognitive and physical activity and dementia: a 44-year longitudinal population study of women. *Neurology.* 2019;92(12):e1322–e1330. doi: 10.1212/WNL.0000000000007021. Epub 2019 Feb 20.

Nauman J, Khan MAB, Joyner MJ. Walking in the fast lane: high-intensity walking for improved fitness and health outcomes. *Mayo Clin Proc.* 2019;94(12):2378–2380. doi: 10.1016/j.mayocp.2019.10.020

Ning K, Zhao L, Matloff W, Sun F, Toga AW. Association of relative brain age with tobacco smoking, alcohol consumption, and genetic variants. *Sci Rep.* 2020;10(1):10. doi: 10.1038/s41598-019-56089-4

Nyberg ST, Singh-Manoux A, Pentti J, et al. Association of healthy lifestyle with years lived without major chronic diseases. *JAMA Intern Med.* 2020;180(5):760–768. doi: 10.1001/jamainternmed.2020.0618

Ogden CL, Fryar CD, Martin CB, et al. Trends in obesity prevalence by race and Hispanic origin: 1999–2000 to 2017–2018. *J Am Med Assoc.* 2020;324(12):1208–1210. doi: 10.1001/jama.2020.14590

Petersen RC, Joyner MJ, Jack CR Jr. Cardiorespiratory fitness and brain volumes. *Mayo Clin Proc.* 2020;95(1):6–8. doi: 10.1016/j.mayocp.2019.11.011

Rêgo ML, Cabral DA, Costa EC, Fontes EB. Physical exercise for individuals with hypertension: it is time to emphasize its benefits on the brain and cognition. *Clin Med Insights Cardiol.* 2019;13:1179546819839411. doi: 10.1177/1179546819839411

Roberts RO, Cha RH, Mielke MM, et al. Risk and protective factors for cognitive impairment in persons aged 85 years and older. *Neurology.* 2015;84(18):1854–1861. doi: 10.1212/WNL.0000000000001537. Epub 2015 Apr 8.

Smith PJ, Blumenthal JA, Hoffman BM, et al. Aerobic exercise and neurocognitive performance: a meta-analytic review of randomized controlled trials. *Psychosom Med.* 2010;72(3):239–252. doi: 10.1097/PSY.0b013e3181d14633. Epub 2010 Mar 11.

Tarumi T, Rossetti H, Thomas BP, et al. Exercise training in amnestic mild cognitive impairment: a one-year randomized controlled trial. *J Alzheimers Dis.* 2019;71(2):421–433. doi: 10.3233/JAD-181175

Tian Q, Resnick SM, Mielke MM, et al. Association of dual decline in memory and gait speed with risk for dementia among adults older than 60 years: a multicohort individual-level meta-analysis. *JAMA Netw Open.* 2020 Feb 5;3(2):e1921636. doi: 10.1001/jamanetworkopen.2019.21636

Walach H, Loef M. Towards primary prevention of Alzheimers disease. *Am J Alzheimers Dis.* 2012;1:1–28. doi: 10.7726/AJAD.2012.1001

Weuve J, Kang JH, Manson JE, Breteler MM, Ware JH, Grodstein F. Physical activity, including walking, and cognitive function in older women. *J Am Med Assoc.* 2004;292(12):1454–1461. doi: 10.1001/jama.292.12.1454

Wittfeld K, Jochem C, Dörr M, et al. Cardiorespiratory fitness and gray matter volume in the temporal, frontal, and cerebellar regions in the general population. *Mayo Clin Proc.* 2020;95(1):44–56. doi: 10.1016/j.mayocp.2019.05.030

Yaffe K, Hoang TD, Byers AL, Barnes DE, Friedl KE. Lifestyle and health-related risk factors and risk of cognitive aging among older veterans. *Alzheimers Dement.* 2014;10(3 Suppl):S111–S121. doi: 10.1016/j.jalz.2014.04.010

Zhu N, Jacobs DR Jr, Schreiner PJ, et al. Cardiorespiratory fitness and cognitive function in middle age: the CARDIA study. *Neurology.* 2014;82(15):1339–1346. doi: 10.1212/WNL.0000000000000310. Epub 2014 Apr 2.

## Chapter 6. Sleeping, Breathing, Breathing while Sleeping

Ahuja S, Chen RK, Kam K, Pettibone WD, Osorio RS, Varga AW. Role of normal sleep and sleep apnea in human memory processing. *Nat Sci Sleep.* 2018;10:255–269. doi: 10.2147/NSS.S125299

Ancoli-Israel S, Palmer BW, Cooke JR, et al. Cognitive effects of treating obstructive sleep apnea in Alzheimer's disease: a randomized controlled study. *J Am Geriatr Soc.* 2008; 56(11): 2076–2081. doi: 10.1007/s11325-021-02320-4

Andre C, Rehel S, Kuhn E, et al. Association of sleep-disordered breathing with Alzheimer disease biomarkers in community-dwelling older adults: a secondary analysis of a randomized clinical trial. *JAMA Neurol.* 2020;77(6):716–724. doi: 10.1001/jamaneurol.2020.0311

Ayalon L, Ancoli-Israel S, Drummond SPA. Obstructive sleep apnea and age: a double insult to brain function? *Am J Respir Crit Care Med.* 2010;182:413–419. doi: 10.1164/rccm.200912-1805OC

Bubu OM, Andrade AG, Umasabor-Bubu OQ, et al. Obstructive sleep apnea, cognition and Alzheimer's disease: a systematic review integrating three decades of multidisciplinary research. *Sleep Med Rev.* 2020; 50:101250. doi: 10.1016/j .smrv.2019.101250

Bubu OM, Brannick M, Mortimer J, et al. Sleep, cognitive impairment, and Alzheimer's disease: a systematic review and meta-analysis. *Sleep.* 2017;40(1). doi: 10.1093/sleep/zsw032

Bubu OM, Pirraglia E, Andrade AG, et al. Obstructive sleep apnea and longitudinal Alzheimer's disease biomarker changes. *Sleep.* 2019;42(6):zsz048. doi: 10.1093/sleep/zsz048

Castronovo V, Canessa N, Ferini Strami L, et al. Brain activation changes before and after PAP treatment in obstructive sleep apnea. *Sleep.* 2009;32(9)1161–1172.

Champagne KA, Kimoff RJ, Barriga PC, Schwartzman K. Sleep disordered breathing in women of childbearing age & during pregnancy. *Indian J Med Res.* 2010; 131:285–301. doi: 10.1097/ogx.0000000000000052

Chen HL, Lin HC, Lu CH, et al. Systemic inflammation and alterations to cerebral blood flow in obstructive sleep apnea. *J Sleep Res.* 2017; 26:789–798. doi: 10.1111/jsr.12553

Chirinos JA, Gurubhagavatula I, Teff K, et al. CPAP, weight loss, or both for obstructive sleep apnea. *N Eng J Med.* 2014;370:265–275. doi: 10.1056/nejm OA1306187

Clionsky E, Clionsky M. A case of apparently reversed Alzheimer's disease. Poster presented at: 2012 Alzheimer's Association International Conference (AAIC2012); July 19, 2012; Vancouver, Canada.

Clionsky M, Clionsky E. Dementia and the brain-breathing connection. *J Alzheimers Dis Parkinsonism.* 2016;6:6. doi: 10.4172/2161-0460.1000e135

Fleming WE, Holty JEC, Bogan RK, et al. Use of blood biomarkers to screen for obstructive sleep apnea. *Nat Sci Sleep.* 2018;10:159–67. doi: 10.2147/NSS .S164488

Hesselbacher S, Aiyer AA, Surani SR, Suleman AA, Varon J. A study to assess the relationship between attention deficit hyperactivity disorder and obstructive sleep apnea in adults. *Cureus.* 2019;11(10):e5979. doi: 10.7759/cureus.5979

Irwin MR, Vitiello MV. Implications of sleep disturbance and inflammation for Alzheimer's disease dementia. *Lancet Neurol.* 2019;18(3):296–306. doi: 10.1016 /S1474-4422(18)30450-2. Epub 2019 Jan 17.

Kim H, Joo EY, Suh S, Kim JH, Kim ST, Hong SB. Effects of long-term treatment on brain volume in patients with obstructive apnea syndrome. *Hum Brain Mapp.* 2016;37:395–409. doi: 10.1002/hbm.23038

Kirsch DB, Yang H, Maslow AL, Stolzenbach M, McCall A. Association of positive airway pressure use with acute care utilization. *J Clin Sleep Med.* 2019;15(9):1243–1250. doi: 10.5664/jcsm.7912

Komaroff AL. Does sleep flush wastes from the brain? *J Am Med Assoc.* 2021 May 17. doi: 10.1001/jama.2021.5631. Epub ahead of print.

Leng Y, McEvoy CT, Allen IE, Yaffe K. Association of sleep-disordered breathing with cognitive function and risk of cognitive impairment: a systematic review and meta-analysis. *JAMA Neurol.* 2017; 74(10):1237–1245. doi: 10.1001 /jamaneurol.2017.2180

Liquori C, Mercuri NB, Izzi F, et al. Obstructive sleep apnea is associated with early but possibly modifiable Alzheimer's disease biomarkers changes. *Sleep,* 2017;40(5):zsx011. doi: 10.1007/s11325-021-02320-4

Marchi NA, Ramponi C, Hirotsu C, et al. Mean oxygen saturation during sleep is related to specific brain atrophy pattern. *Ann Neurol*. 2020;87:921–930. doi: 10.1002/ana.25728

McMillan A, Morrell MJ. Sleep disordered breathing at the extremes of age: the elderly. *Breathe*. 2016;12:50–60. doi: 10.1183/20734735.003216

Osorio RS, Gumb T, Pirraglia E, et al. Sleep-disordered breathing advances cognitive decline in the elderly. *Neurology*. 2015;84:1964–1971. doi: 10.1212/WNL .0000000000001566. Epub 2015 Apr 15.

Proskovec AL, Rezich MT, O'Neill J, et al. Association of epigenetic metrics of biological age with cortical thickness. *JAMA Netw Open*. 2020; 3(9):e2015428. doi: 10.1001/jamanetworkopen.2020.15428

Reynolds CF III, Kupfer D, Taska LS, et al. Sleep apnea in Alzheimer's dementia: correlation with mental deterioration. *J Clin Psychiatry*. 1985;46(7):257–261.

Richards KC, Gooneratne N, Dicicco B, et al. CPAP adherence may slow 1-year cognitive decline in older adults with mild cognitive impairment and apnea. *J Am Geriatr Soc*. 2019;67:558–564. doi: 10.1111/jgs.15758

Robbins R, Quan SF, Weaver MD, Bormes G, Barger LK, Czeisler CA. Examining sleep deficiency and disturbance and their risk for incident dementia and all-cause mortality in older adults across 5 years in the United States. *Aging* (Albany NY). 2021 Feb 11;13(3):3254–3268. doi: 10.18632/aging.202591. Epub 2021 Feb 11.

Senaratna CV, Perret JL, Lodge CJ, et al. Prevalence of obstructive sleep apnea in the general population: a systematic review. *Sleep Med Rev*. 2017;34:70–81. doi: 10.1016/j.smrv.2016.07.002

Shi L, Chen SJ, Ma MY, et al. Sleep disturbances increase the risk of dementia: a systematic review and meta-analysis. *Sleep Med Rev*. 2018;40:4–16. Epub 2017 Jul 6. doi: 10.1016/j.smrv.2017.06.010

Shokri-Kojori E, Wang GJ, Wiers CE, et al. β-Amyloid accumulation in the human brain after one night of sleep deprivation. *Proc Natl Acad Sci USA*. 2018;115(17):4483–4488. doi: 10.1073/pnas.1721694115. Epub 2018 Apr 9.

Somers VK, White D, Amin R, et al. Sleep apnea and cardiovascular disease. *J Am Coll Cardiol*. 2008;52(8):686–717. doi: 10.1161/CIRCULATIONAHA.107.189375. Epub 2008 Aug 25.

Sun X, He G, Qing H, et al. Hypoxia facilitates Alzheimer's disease pathogenesis by up-regulating BACE1 gene expression. *PNAS*. 2006;103(49):18727–18732. doi: 10.1073/pnas.0606298103

Tsai M-S, Li H-Y, Huang C-G, et al. Risk of Alzheimer's disease in obstructive sleep apnea patients with or without treatment: real-world evidence. *Laryngoscope.* 2020;130: 2292–2298. doi: 10.1002/lary.28558

Van Dongen HP, Maislin G, Mullington JM, Dinges DF. The cumulative cost of additional wakefulness: dose-response effects on neurobehavioral functions and sleep physiology from chronic sleep restriction and total sleep deprivation. *Sleep.* 2003;26(2):117–126. doi: 10.1093/sleep/26.2.117. Erratum in: *Sleep.* 2004 Jun 15;27(4):600.

Veasey SC, Rosen IM. Obstructive sleep apnea in adults. *N Eng J Med.* 2019;380:1442–49. doi: 10.1056/NEJMcp1816152

Wang Y, Cheng C, Moelter S, et al. One year of continuous positive airway pressure adherence improves cognition in older adults with mild apnea and mild cognitive impairment. *Nurs Res.* 2020;69(2):157–164. doi: 10.1097/NNR .0000000000000420

Wu J, Gu M, Chen S, et al. Factors related to pediatric obstructive sleep apnea-hypopnea syndrome in children with attention deficit hyperactivity disorder in different age groups. *Medicine.* 2017;96(42):e8281. doi: 10.1097 /MD.0000000000008281

Xie L, Kang H, Xu Q, et al. Sleep drives metabolite clearance from the adult brain. *Science.* 2013; 342(6156):373–377. doi: 10.1126/science.1241224

Yaffe C, Laffan AM, Harrison SL, et al. Sleep disordered breathing, hypoxia, and risk of mild cognitive impairment and dementia in older women. *J Am Med Assoc.* 2011;306(6):613–619. doi: 10.1001/jama.2011.1115

Youssef NA, Ege M, Angly SS, Strauss JL, Marx CE. Is obstructive sleep apnea associated with ADHD? *Ann Clin Psychiatry.* 2011;23(3):213–224.

Zetterberg H, Mortberg E, Song L, et al. Hypoxia due to cardiac arrest induces a time-dependent increase in serum amyloid $\beta$ levels in humans. *PLoS One.* 2011;6(12):e28263. doi: 10.1371/journal.pone.0028263

## Chapter 7. Metabolic and Vitamin Deficiencies

Balion C, Griffith LE, Strifler L, et al. Vitamin D, cognition, and dementia: a systematic review and meta-analysis. *Neurology.* 2012;79(13);1397–1405. doi: 10.1212/WNL.0b013e31826c197f

Bauer SR, Kapoor A, Rath M, Thomas SA. What is the role of supplementation with ascorbic acid, zinc, vitamin D, or N-acetylcysteine for prevention or treatment of COVID-19? *Cleve Clin J Med.* 2020 Jun 8. doi: 10.3949/ccjm.87a.ccc046

Beydoun MA, Beydoun HA, Gamaldo AA, Teel A, Zonderman AB, Wang Y. Epidemiologic studies of modifiable factors associated with cognition and dementia: systematic review and meta-analysis. *BMC Public Health.* 2014;14(643). doi: 10.1186/1471-2458-14-643

Bjelakovic G, Gluud L, Nikolova D, et al. Vitamin D supplementation for prevention of mortality in adults. *Cochrane Database Syst Rev.* 2014,1(CD007470). doi: 10.1002/14651858.CD007470.pub3

Blasko I, Hinterberger M, Kemmlesr G, et al. Conversion from mild cognitive impairment to dementia: influence of folic acid and vitamin B12 use in the vita cohort. *J Nutr Health Aging.* 2012;16(8):687–694. doi: 10.1007/s12603-012-0051-y

Buell JS, Dawson-Hughes B, Scott TM, et al. 25-hydroxyvitamin D, dementia, and cerebrovascular pathology in elders receiving home services. *Neurology.* 2010;74(1):18–26. doi: 10.1212/WNL.0b013e3181beecb7. Epub 2009 Nov 25.

Camaschella C. Iron-deficiency anemia. *N Eng J Med.* 2015;372(19):1832–1843. doi: 10.1056/NEJMra1401038

Clarke R, Smith AD, Jobst KA, Refsum H, Sutton L, Ueland PM. Folate, vitamin B12, and serum total homocysteine levels in confirmed Alzheimer disease. *Arch Neurol.* 1998;55(11):1449–1455. doi: 10.1001/archneur.55.11.1449

Clemens TL. Vitamin B12 deficiency and bone health. *N Eng J Med.* 2014;371:963–964. doi: 10.1056/NEJMcibr1407247

Council for Responsible Nutrition. Dietary supplement use reaches all time high. www.crnusa.org/newsroom/dietary-supplement-use-reaches-all-time-high#

Dash P, Hergenroeder G, Jeter C, Choi H, Kobori N, Moore A. Traumatic brain injury alters methionine metabolism: implications for pathophysiology. *Front Syst Neurosci.* 2016.10:36. doi: 10.3389/fnsys.2016.00036

Ebly EM, Schaefer JP, Campbell NR, Hogan DB. Folate status, vascular disease and cognition in elderly Canadians. *Age Ageing.* 1998;27(4):485–491. doi: 10.1093/ageing/27.4.485

Ganji V, Kafai MR. Population references for plasma total homocysteine concentrations for U.S. children and adolescents in the post-folic acid fortification era. *J Nutr.* 2005;135(9):2253–2256. doi: 10.1093/jn/135.9.2253

Geisel T, Martin J, Schulze B, et al. An etiologic profile of anemia in 405 geriatric patients. *Anemia*. 2014;932486. doi: 10.1155/2014/942486. Epub 2014 Feb 23.

Giles WH, Croft JB, Greenlund KJ, Ford ES, Kittner SJ. Total homocyst(e)ine concentration and the likelihood of nonfatal stroke: results from the Third National Health and Nutrition Examination Survey, 1988–1994. *Stroke*. 1998;29(12):2473–2477. doi: 10.1161/01.str.29.12.2473

Goss AM, Gower B, Soleymani T, et al. Effects of weight loss during a very low carbohydrate diet on specific adipose tissue depots and insulin sensitivity in older adults with obesity: a randomized clinical trial. *Nutri Metab*. 2020;17(64). doi: 10.1186/s12986-020-00481-9

Hannibal L, Lysne V, Bjørke-Monsen A-L, et al. Biomarkers and algorithms for the diagnosis of vitamin B12 deficiency. *Front Mol Biosci*. 2016;3.27. doi: 10.3389/fmolb.2016.00027

Haan MN, Miller JW, Aiello AE, et al. Homocysteine, B vitamins, and the incidence of dementia and cognitive impairment: results from the Sacramento Area Latino Study on Aging. *Am J Clin Nutr*. 2007;85(2):511–517. doi: 10.1093/ajcn/85.2.511

Harkin A. Muscling in on depression. *N Eng J Med*. 2014;371:2333–2334. doi: 10.1056/NEJMcibr1411568

Hicks GE, Shardell M, Miller RR, et al. Associations between vitamin D status and pain in older adults: The Invecchiare in Chianti Study. *J Am Geriatr Soc*. 2008;56:785–791. doi: 10.1111/j.1532–5415.2008.01644.x

Ho PI, Ortiz D, Rogers E, Shea TB. Multiple aspects of homocysteine neurotoxicity: glutamate excitotoxicity, kinase hyperactivation and DNA damage. *J Neurosci Res*. 2002;70(5):694–702. doi: 10.1002/jnr.10416

Holick MF. High prevalence of vitamin D inadequacy and implications for health. *Mayo Clin Proc*. 2006; 81(3):353–373. doi: 10.4065/81.3.353

Holland TM, Agarwal P, Wang Y, et al. Dietary flavonols and risk of Alzheimer dementia. *Neurology*. 2020;94(16):e1749–e1756; doi: 10.1212/WNL.0000000000008981

Jáuregui-Lobera I. Iron deficiency and cognitive functions. *Neuropsychiatr Dis Treat*. 2014;10(10):2087–2095. doi: 10.2147/NDT.S72491

Jochemsen HM, Kloppenborg RP, de Groot LC, et al. Homocysteine, progression of ventricular enlargement, and cognitive decline: the Second Manifestations of Arterial Disease-Magnetic Resonance Study. *Alzheimers Dement*. 2013;9(3):302–309. doi: 10.1016/j.jalz.2011.11.008. Epub 2012 Aug 3.

Kang JH, Cook N, Manson J, Buring JE, Albert CM, Grodstein F. A trial of B vitamins and cognitive function among women at high risk of cardiovascular disease. *Am J Clin Nutr.* 2008;88(6):1602–1610. doi: 10.3945/ajcn.2008.26404

Köhnke C, Herrmann M, Berger K. Associations of major depressive disorder and
related clinical characteristics with 25-hydroxyvitamin D levels in middle-aged
adults. *Nutr Neurosci.* 2020;9:1–10. doi: 10.1080/1028415X.2020.1843892. Epub
ahead of print.

Lipton SA, Kim WK, Choi YB, et al. Neurotoxicity associated with dual actions of
homocysteine at the N-methyl-D-aspartate receptor. *Proc Natl Acad Sci USA.*
1997;94(11):5923–5928. doi: 10.1073/pnas.94.11.5923

Llewellyn DJ, Lang IA, Langa KM, et al. Vitamin D and risk of cognitive decline
in elderly persons. *Arch Intern Med.* 2010;170(13):1135–1141. doi: 10.1001
/archinternmed.2010.173

Malinow MR, Bostom AG, Krauss RM. Homocyst(e)ine, diet, and cardiovascular
diseases: a statement for healthcare professionals from the Nutrition Com-
mittee, American Heart Association. *Circulation.* 1999 Jan 5–12;99(1):178–182.
doi: 10.1161/01.cir.99.1.178

Masoumi A, Goldenson B, Ghirmai S, et al. 1alpha,25-dihydroxyvitamin D3 inter-
acts with curcuminoids to stimulate amyloid-beta clearance by macrophages of
Alzheimer's disease patients. *J Alzheimers Dis.* 2009;17(3):703–717. doi: 10.3233
/JAD-2009-1080

Mizwicki MT, Menegaz D, Zhang J, et al. Genomic and nongenomic signaling
induced by 1α,25(OH)2-vitamin D3 promotes the recovery of amyloid-β phago-
cytosis by Alzheimer's disease macrophages. *J Alzheimers Dis.* 2012;29(1):51–62.
doi: 10.3233/JAD-2012-110560

Mujica-Parodi LR, Amgalan A, Sultan SF, et al. Diet modulates brain network
stability, a biomarker for brain aging, in young adults. *Proc Natl Acad Sci.*
2020;117(11):6170–6177; doi: 10.1073/pnas.1913042117

Okereke OI, Reynolds CF, Mischoulon D, et al. Effect of long-term vitamin D3 supplementation vs placebo on risk of depression or clinically relevant depressive
symptoms and on change in mood scores: a randomized clinical trial. *J Am
Med Assoc.* 2020;324(5):471–480. doi: 10.1001/jama.2020.10224

Paillusson S, Stoica R, Gómez-Suaga P, et al. There's something wrong with my
MAM: the ER–mitochondria axis and neurodegenerative diseases. *Trends Neurosci.* 2016;39(3):146–157. doi: 10.1016/j.tins.2016.01.008

Pilling LC, Jones LC, Masoli JAH, et al. Low vitamin D levels and risk of incident delirium in 351,000 older UK Biobank participants. *J Am Geriatr Soc.* 2021;69(2):365–372. doi: 10.1111/jgs.16853. Epub 2020 Oct 5.

Prins ND, den Heijer T, Hofman A, et al. Homocysteine and cognitive function in the elderly: the Rotterdam Scan Study. *Neurology.* 2002;59(9):1375–1380. doi: 10.1212/01.WNL.0000032494.05619.93

Ravaglia G, Forti P, Maioli F, et al. Homocysteine and folate as risk factors for dementia and Alzheimer disease. *Am J Clin Nutr.* 2005;82(3):636–643. doi: 10.1093/ajcn/82.3.636

Regland B, McCaddon A. Alzheimer's amyloidopathy: an alternative aspect. *J Alzheimers Dis.* 2019;68(2):483–488. doi: 10.3233/JAD-181007

Rodgers GP, Collins FS. Precision nutrition: the answer to "what to eat to stay healthy." *J Am Med Assoc.* 2020;324(8):735–736. doi: 10.1001/jama.2020.13601

Salminen A, Kauppinen A, Suuronen T, Kaarniranta K, Ojala J. ER stress in Alzheimer's disease: a novel neuronal trigger for inflammation and Alzheimer's pathology. *J Neuroinflammation.* 2009;41. doi: 10.1186/1742-2094-6-41

Seshadri S, Beiser A, Selhub J, et al. Plasma homocysteine as a risk factor for dementia and Alzheimer's disease. *N Eng J Med.* 2002;346(7):476–483. doi: 10.1056/NEJMoa011613

Slinin Y, Paudel ML, Taylor BC, et al. 25-Hydroxyvitamin D levels and cognitive performance and decline in elderly men. *Neurology.* 2010;74(1):33–41. doi: 10.1212/wnl.0b013e3181c7197b

Smith AD, Refsum H, Bottiglieri T, et al. Homocysteine and dementia: an international consensus statement. *J Alzheimers Dis.* 2018;62(2):561–570. doi: 10.3233/JAD-171042

Smith AD, Smith SM, de Jager CA, et al. Homocysteine-lowering by B vitamins slows the rate of accelerated brain atrophy in mild cognitive impairment: a randomized controlled trial. *PLoS One.* 2010. doi: 10.1371/journal.pone.0012244

Spedding S. Vitamins are more funky than Casimir thought. *Australas Med J.* 2013;6(2):104–106. doi: 10.4066/AMJ.2013.1588

Taheri S, Lin L, Austin D, Young T, Mignot E. Short sleep duration is associated with reduced leptin, elevated ghrelin, and increased body mass index. *PLOS Medicine,* 2004;1,e62. doi: 10.1371/journal.pmed.0010062

Tezapsidis N, Johnston JM, Smith MA, et al. Leptin: a novel therapeutic strategy for Alzheimer's disease. *J Alzheimers Dis*. 2009;16(4):731–740. doi: 10.3233 /jad-2009-1021

Tucker KL, Qiao N, Scott T, Rosenberg I, Spiro A III. High homocysteine and low B vitamins predict cognitive decline in aging men: the Veterans Affairs Normative Aging Study. *Am J Clin Nutr*. 2005;82(3):627–635. doi: 10.1093/ajcn.82.3.627

Wish JB. Assessing iron status: beyond serum ferritin and transferrin saturation. *Clin J Am Soc Nephrol*. 2006 Sep;1 Suppl 1:S4–S8. doi: 10.2215/CJN.01490506

Xu W, Tan L, Wang HF, et al. Meta-analysis of modifiable risk factors for Alzheimer's disease. *J Neurol Neurosurg Psychiatry*. 2015;86(12):1299–1306. doi: 10.1136/jnnp-2015-310548. Epub 2015 Aug 20.

Yassine HN, Braskie MN, Mack WJ, et al. Association of docosahexaenoic acid supplementation with Alzheimer disease stage in apolipoprotein E ε4 carriers: a review. *JAMA Neurol*. 2017;74(3):339–347. doi: 10.1001/jamaneurol.2016.4899

Zhao C, Tsapanou A, Manly J, Schupf, N, Brickman AM, Gu, Y. Vitamin D intake is associated with dementia risk in the Washington Heights–Inwood Columbia Aging Project (WHICAP). *Alzheimers Dement*. 2020;16:1393–1401. doi: 10.1002 /alz.12096

## Chapter 8. Alcohol, Drugs, and Medications

Alexander CM, Seifert HA, Blouin RT, Conrad PF, Gross JB. Diphenhydramine enhances the interaction of hypercapnic and hypoxic ventilatory drive. *Anesthesiology*. 1994;80:789–795.

Boeuf-Cazou O, Bongue B, Ansiau D, Marquie J-C, Lapeyre-Mestre M. Impact of long-term benzodiazepine use on cognitive functioning in young adults: the VISAT cohort. *Eur J Clin Pharmacol*. 2011;67:1045. doi: 10.1007/s00228-011 -1047-y

Campbell NL, Holden R, Boustani MA. Preventing Alzheimer disease by deprescribing anticholinergic medications. *JAMA Intern Med*. 2019;179(8):1093–1094. doi: 10.1001/jamainternmed.2019.0676

Cohen PA, Avula B, Wang YH, Zakharevich I, Khan I. Five unapproved drugs found in cognitive enhancement supplements. *Neurol Clin Pract*. 2021;11(3):e303–e307. doi: 10.1212/CPJ.0000000000000960

Coupland CAC, Hill T, Dening T, Morriss R, Moore M, Hippisley-Cox J. Anticholinergic drug exposure and the risk of dementia: a nested case-control

study. *JAMA Intern Med.* 2019;179(8):1084–1093. doi: 10.1001/jamaintern
med.2019.0677

Crowe S, Stranks E. The residual medium and long-term cognitive effects of
benzodiazepine use: an updated meta-analysis. *Arch Clin Neuropsychol.*
2018;33:901–911. doi: 10.1093/arclin/acx120

D'Amico G, deFranchis R, Dell'Era A, eds. *National history and stages of cir-
rhosis and variceal hemorrhage.* Springer Science+Business Media; 2014.
doi: 10.1007/978-1-4939-0002-2_2

Esser MB, Sherk A, Liu Y, et al. Deaths and years of potential life lost from excessive alcohol use—United States, 2011–2015. *Morbidity and Mortality Weekly
Report.* 2020;69:981–987. doi: 10.15585/mmwr.mm6930a1

Flippo TS, Holder WD. Neurologic degeneration associated with nitrous
oxide anesthesia in patients with vitamin B12 deficiency. *Arch Surg.*
1993;128(12):1391–1395. doi: 10.1001/archsurg.1993.01420240099018

Gray SL, Anderson ML, Dublin S, et al. Cumulative use of strong anticholinergics and incident dementia: a prospective cohort study. *JAMA Intern Med.*
2015;175(3):401–407. doi: 10.1001/jamainternmed.2014.7663

Harper CG, Giles M, Finlay-Jones R. Clinical signs in the Wernicke-Korsakoff
complex: a retrospective analysis of 131 cases diagnosed at necropsy. *J Neurol
Neurosurg Psychiatry.* 1986;49:341–345.

He Q, Chen X, Wu T, Li L, Fei X. Risk of dementia in long-term benzodiazepine
users: evidence from a meta-analysis of observational studies. *J Clin Neurol.*
2019;15(1):9–19. doi: 10.3988/jcn.2019.15.1.9. Epub 2018 Oct 26.

Islam MM, Iqbal U, Walther B, et al. Benzodiazepine use and risk of dementia in
the elderly population: a systematic review and meta-analysis. *Neuroepidemiol-
ogy.* 2016;47:181–191. doi: 10.1159/000454881

Kim JW, Lee DY, Lee BC, et al. Alcohol and cognition in the elderly: a review.
*Psychiatry Investig.* 2012;9:8–16. doi: 10.4306/pi.2012.9.1.8

Kivimäki M, Singh-Manoux A, Batty GD, et al. Association of alcohol-induced loss
of consciousness and overall alcohol consumption with risk for dementia.
*JAMA Netw Open.* 2020;3(9):e2016084. doi: 10.1001/jamanetworkopen.2020
.16084

National Institute on Alcohol Abuse and Alcoholism. *Alcohol facts and statistics.*
https://www.niaaa.nih.gov/publications/brochures-and-fact-sheets/alcohol
-facts-and-statistics

Oscar-Berman M, Marinkovic K. Alcoholism and the brain: an overview. *Alcohol Res Health.* 2003;27(2):125–133.

Paterniti S, Dufouil C, Alpérovitch A. Long-term benzodiazepine use and cognitive decline in the elderly: the epidemiology of vascular aging study. *J Clin Psychopharmacol.* 2002;22(3):285–293.

Raphael KC, Matuja SS, Shen NT, Liwa AC, Jaka H. Hepatic encephalopathy; prevalence, precipitating factors and challenges of management in a resource-limited setting. *J Gastrointest Digest Syst.* 2016;6(3):441. doi: 10.4172/2161-069X.1000441

Rösner S, Soyka M, Hajak G, Wehrle R, Englbrecht C. Eszopiclone for insomnia. *Cochrane Database System Rev.* 2013;8(CD010703). doi: 10.1002/14651858 .CD010703

Rudolph JL, Salow MJ, Angelini MC, McGlinchey RE. The anticholinergic risk scale and anticholinergic adverse effects in older persons. *Arch Intern Med.* 2008;168(5):508–513. doi: 10.1001/archinternmed.2007.106

Sabia S, Elbaz A, Britton A, Bell S, Dugravot A, Shipley M, Kivimaki M, Singh-Manoux A. Alcohol consumption and cognitive decline in early old age. *Neurology.* 2014;82(4):332–339. doi: 10.1212/WNL.0000000000000063. Epub 2014 Jan 15.

Sacks O, Shulman M. Steroid dementia: An overlooked diagnosis? *Neurology.* 2005;64:707–709.

Schwarzinger M, Pollock BG, Hasan OSM, Dufouil C, Rehm J; QalyDays Study Group. Contribution of alcohol use disorders to the burden of dementia in France 2008–13: a nationwide retrospective cohort study. *Lancet Public Health.* 2018;3(3):e124–132. doi: 10.1016/S2468-2667(18)30022-7. Epub 2018 Feb 21.

Topiwala A, Allan CL, Valkanova V, et al. Moderate alcohol consumption as risk factor for adverse brain outcomes and cognitive decline: longitudinal cohort study. *BMJ.* 2017;357:j2353. doi: 10.1136/bmj.j2353

Vilstrup H, Amodio P, Bajaj J, et al. Hepatic encephalopathy in chronic liver disease: 2014 practice guideline by the American Association for the Study of Liver Diseases and the European Association for the Study of the Liver. *Hepatology.* 2014;60(2):715–735. doi: 10.1002/hep.27210. Epub 2014 Jul 8.

Weigand AJ, Bondi MW, Thomas KR, et al. Association of anticholinergic medications and AD biomarkers with incidence of MCI among cognitively normal older adults. *Neurology.* 2020;95(16) e2295–e2304. doi: 10.1212/WNL .0000000000010643

Wein C, Koch H, Popp B, Oehler G, Schauder P. Minimal hepatic encephalopathy impairs fitness to drive. *Hepatology*. 2004;39(3):739–745. doi: 10.1002/hep.20095

Wright JD, Cogan JC, Huang Y, et al. Association of new perioperative benzodiazepine use with persistent benzodiazepine use. *JAMA Netw Open*. 2021;4(6):e2112478. doi: 10.1001/jamanetworkopen.2021.12478

Wu CS, Ting TT, Wang SC, Chang IS, Lin KM. Effect of benzodiazepine discontinuation on dementia risk. *Am J Geriatr Psychiatry*. 2011;19(2):151–159. doi: 10.1097/JGP.0b013e3181e049ca

Zhang R, Shen L, Miles T, et al. Association of low to moderate alcohol drinking with cognitive functions from middle to older age among US adults. *JAMA Netw Open*. 2020;3(6):e207922. doi: 10.1001/jamanetworkopen.2020.7922

## Chapter 9. Sensory and Emotional Factors That Amplify Dementia Risk

Bamia C, Trichopoulou A, Trichopoulos D. Age at retirement and mortality in a general population sample: the Greek EPIC study. *Am J Epidemiol*. 2008;167(5):561–569. doi: 10.1093/aje/kwm337. Epub 2007 Dec 3.

Bialystok E. Bilingualism: pathway to cognitive reserve. *Trends Cogn Sci*. 2021;25(5):355–364. doi: 10.1016/j.tics.2021.02.003. Epub 2021 Mar 23.

Biddle KD, Jacobs HIL, d'Oleire Uquillas F, et al. Associations of widowhood and β-amyloid with cognitive decline in cognitively unimpaired older adults. *JAMA Netw Open*. 2020;3(2):e200121. doi: 10.1001/jamanetworkopen.2020.0121

Brenowitz WD, Besser LM, Kukull WA, Keene CD, Glymour MM, Yaffe K. Clinician-judged hearing impairment and associations with neuropathologic burden. *Neurology*. 2020;95(12):e1640–e1649; doi: 10.1212/WNL .0000000000010575

Bubbico G, Chiacchiaretta P, Parenti M, et al. Effects of second language learning on the plastic aging brain: functional connectivity, cognitive decline, and reorganization. *Front Neurosci*. 2019;13:423. doi: 10.3389/fnins.2019.00423. eCollection 2019.

Deal JA, Goman AM, Albert MS, et al. Hearing treatment for reducing cognitive decline: design and methods of the Aging and Cognitive Health Evaluation in Elders randomized controlled trial. *Alzheimer Dement*. 2018;4:499–507. doi: 10.1016/j.trci.2018.08.007

Dekhtyar S, Marseglia A, Xu W, Darin-Mattsson A, Wang HX, Fratiglioni L. Genetic risk of dementia mitigated by cognitive reserve: a cohort study. *Ann of Neurol.* 2019;86(1):68–78. doi: 10.1002/ana.25501. Epub 2019 May 22.

Devere R. Music and dementia: an overview. *Pract Neurol.* 2017. https://practical neurology.com/articles/2017-june/music-and-dementia-an-overview/pdf

Diniz BS, Butters MA, Albert SM, Dew MA, Reynolds CF III. Late-life depression and risk of vascular dementia and Alzheimer's disease: systematic review and meta-analysis of community-based cohort studies. *Br J Psychiatry.* 2013;202(5):329–335. doi: 10.1192/bjp.bp.112.118307

Ehrlich JR, Goldstein J, Swenor BK, Whitson H, Langa KM, Veliz P. Addition of vision impairment to a life-course model of potentially modifiable dementia risk factors in the US. *JAMA Neurol.* 2022 Jun 1;79(6):623–626. doi: 10.1001 /jamaneurol.2022.0723. Erratum in: *JAMA Neurol.* 2022 Jun 1;79(6):634.

Fancourt D, Steptoe A. Television viewing and cognitive decline in older age: findings from the English Longitudinal Study of Ageing. *Sci Rep.* 2019;9(1):2851. doi: 10.1038/s41598-019-39354-4

Golub JS, Brickman AM, Ciarleglio AJ, Schupf N, Luchsinger JA. Association of subclinical hearing loss with cognitive performance. *JAMA Otolaryngol Head Neck Surg.* 2020 Jan 1;146(1):57–67. doi: 10.1001/jamaoto.2019.3375

Griffiths TD, Lad M, Kumar S, et al. How can hearing loss cause dementia? *Neuron.* 2020;108(3):401–412. doi: 10.1016/j.neuron.2020.08.003. Epub 2020 Aug 31.

Guzzo R, Nalbantian H. Is the gig economy the answer for older workers? May 9, 2019. https://www.brinknews.com/is-the-gig-economy-the-answer-for-older -workers/

Harshfield EL, Pennells L, Schwartz JE, et al. Association between depressive symptoms and incident cardiovascular diseases. *J Am Med Assoc.* 2020;324(23):2396–2405. doi: 10.1001/jama.2020.23068

Hwang PH, Longstreth WT Jr., Brenowitz WD, et al. Dual sensory impairment in older adults and risk of dementia from the GEM Study. *Alzheimers Dement.* 2020;12(1):e12054. doi: 10.1002/dad2.12054

Kable JW, Caulfield MK, Falcone M, et al. No effect of commercial cognitive training on brain activity, choice behavior, or cognitive performance. *J Neurosci.* 2017,37(31):7390–7402. doi: 10.1523/JNEUROSCI.2832-16.2017

Kapasi A, DeCarli C, Schneider JA. Impact of multiple pathologies on the threshold for clinically overt dementia. *Acta Neuropathologica*. 2017;134(2):171–186. doi: 10.1007/s00401-017-1717-7. Epub 2017 May 9.

Karawania H, Jenkins KA, Anderson S. Restoration of sensory input may improve cognitive and neural function. *Neuropsychologia*. 2018;114:203–213. doi: 10.1016/j.neuropsychologia.2018.04.041

Karawania H, Jenkins KA, Anderson S. Neural and behavioral changes after the use of hearing aids. *Clinical Neurophysiol*. 2018;129(6): 1254–1267. doi: 10.1016 /j.clinph.2018.03.024

Li C, Zhang X, Hoffman HJ, Cotch MF, Themann CL, Wilson MR. Hearing impairment associated with depression in US adults, National Health and Nutrition Examination Survey 2005–2010. *JAMA Otolaryngol Head Neck Surg*. 2014;140(4):293–302. doi: 10.1001/jamaoto.2014.42

Lin FR, Albert M. Hearing loss and dementia—who is listening? *Aging Ment Health*. 2014;18:6, 671–673. doi: 10.1080/13607863.2014.915924

Liu H, Zhang Z, Choi SW, Langa KM. Marital status and dementia: evidence from the Health and Retirement Study. *J Gerontol B Psychol Sci Soc Sci*. 2020;75(8):1783–1795. doi: 10.1093/geronb/gbz087

Lozupone M, Sardone R, Panza F. Age-related hearing loss and neuropathologic burden: a step inside the cognitive ear. *Neurology*. 2020; 95(12)511–512. doi: 10.1212/WNL.0000000000010580

Mayeda ER, Mobley TM, Weiss RE, Murchland AR, Berkman LF, Sabbath EL. Association of work-family experience with mid- and late-life memory decline in US women. *Neurology*. 2020;95(23):e3072–e3080. doi: 10.1212 /WNL.0000000000010989. Epub 2020 Nov 4.

Mendez MF, Perryman KM, Pontón MO, Cummings JL. Bilingualism and dementia. *J Neuropsychiatry Clin Neurosci*. 1999;11(3):411–412. doi: 10.1176/jnp.11 .3.411

Piccinni A, Origlia N, Veltri A, et al. Neurodegeneration, β-amyloid and mood disorders: state of the art and future perspectives. *Int J Geriatr Psychiatry*. 2013;28:661-671. doi: 28.10.1002/gps.3879

Rong H, Lai X, Jing R, Wang X, Fang H, Mahmoudi E. Association of sensory impairments with cognitive decline and depression among older adults in China. *JAMA Netw Open*. 2020;3(9):e2014186. doi: 10.1001/jamanetworkopen .2020.14186

Saczynski JS, Beiser A, Seshadri S, Auerbach S, Wolf PA, Au R. Depressive symptoms and risk of dementia: the Framingham Heart Study. *Neurology*. 2010;75:35–41. doi: 10.1212/WNL.0b013e3181e62138

Sindi S, Mangialasche F, Kivipelto M. Advances in the prevention of Alzheimer's disease. *F1000Prime Rep*. 2015;7:50. doi: 10.12703/P7-50

Sundström A, Rönnlund M, Josefsson M. A nationwide Swedish study of age at retirement and dementia risk. *Int J Geriatr Psychiatry*. 2020;35:1243–1249. doi: 10.1002/gps.5363

Tran EM, Stefanick ML, Henderson VW, et al. Association of visual impairment with risk of incident dementia in a women's health initiative population. *JAMA Ophthalmol*. 2020;138(6):624–633. doi: 10.1001/jamaophthalmol.2020.0959

Wuwongse S, Chang RC, Law AC. The putative neurodegenerative links between depression and Alzheimer's disease. *Prog Neurobiol*. 2010;91(4):362–375. doi: 10.1016/j.pneurobio.2010.04.005. Epub 2010 May 2.

Zheng DD, Swenor BK, Christ SL, West SK, Lam BL, Lee DJ. Longitudinal associations between visual impairment and cognitive functioning: the Salisbury Eye Evaluation Study. *JAMA Ophthalmol*. 2018;136(9):989–995. doi: 10.1001/jamaophthalmol.2018.2493

## Chapter 10. Putting It All Together in an Interactive Dementia Risk Model

Kivipelto M, Solomon A, Ahtiluoto S, et al. The Finnish Geriatric Intervention Study to Prevent Cognitive Impairment and Disability (FINGER): study design and progress. *Alzheimers Dement*. 2013;9(6):657–665.

# Index

acetylcholine, 110–11, 112, 131, 151–52

adenosine triphosphate (ATP), 78, 79, 150, 154

Advanced Dementia Treatment protocol, 6–9

aging, as dementia risk factor, 22, 24, 133

airways, in sleep apnea, 9, 81–82, 90, 91, 92, 93–94, 129, 130–31, 198, 199, 204

alcohol consumption, 1, 2, 6, 11, 18, 40, 75, 128, 150, 160; adverse cognitive effects of, 31, 106–9, 127, 132, 158; adverse physical effects of, 92, 105–6; binge drinking, 105, 109; as blackout cause, 107–8, 109, 163–64; evaluation of drinking habits, 144, 155–56, 169; low-to-moderate levels of, 106, 107, 108–9, 170; management of, 161–62, 170; during pregnancy, 51–52; in women, 51–52, 105, 106

alcohol withdrawal, 109, 153

alleles, 48, 49–50, 53–54

alprazolam (Xanax), 109, 153, 169, 178

Alzheimer, Alois, 25, 26, 28, 30, 85, 182

Alzheimer disease, 1, 4, 6, 10, 12, 22, 31, 76, 85, 108, 151–52; biomarkers, 19–20, 39, 41, 88, 90, 121; brain structure changes in, 25–26, 27, 39, 40, 93, 95, 99; diet and, 66–67; drug therapy for, 10, 12, 111, 152; early-onset, 50; as form of dementia, 17, 24, 28, 29; history of, 25–29; information for caregivers about, 12; mid-to-late-stage, 12; "pure," 24; reversal of, 92–95; risk factors for, 31, 49–50, 66, 67, 76, 77, 78, 85, 88, 89, 90, 93, 120; with vascular dementia, 20–21, 24

Alzheimer's Association International Conference, 95

Alzheimer's Disease and Related Disorders Association, 12, 29

Alzheimer's Disease Neuroimaging Initiative (ADNI), 41, 89

American Academy of Neurology, 72, 95

American Board of Psychiatry and Neurology, 5

# HEALTH & WELLNESS BOOKS FROM HOPKINS PRESS

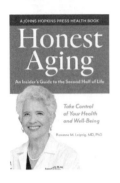
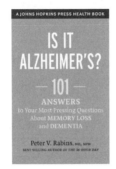
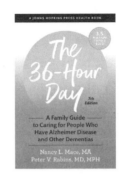
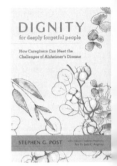

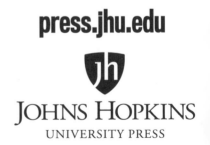